EBOLA IN THE HOMELAND: THE IMPORTANCE OF EFFECTIVE INTERNATIONAL, FEDERAL, STATE, AND LOCAL COORDINATION

FIELD HEARING

BEFORE THE

COMMITTEE ON HOMELAND SECURITY HOUSE OF REPRESENTATIVES

ONE HUNDRED THIRTEENTH CONGRESS

SECOND SESSION

OCTOBER 10, 2014

Serial No. 113–88

Printed for the use of the Committee on Homeland Security

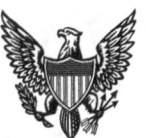

Available via the World Wide Web: http://www.gpo.gov/fdsys/

U.S. GOVERNMENT PUBLISHING OFFICE

93–646 PDF   WASHINGTON : 2015

For sale by the Superintendent of Documents, U.S. Government Publishing Office
Internet: bookstore.gpo.gov   Phone: toll free (866) 512–1800; DC area (202) 512–1800
Fax: (202) 512–2104   Mail: Stop IDCC, Washington, DC 20402–0001

COMMITTEE ON HOMELAND SECURITY

MICHAEL T. MCCAUL, Texas, *Chairman*

LAMAR SMITH, Texas
PETER T. KING, New York
MIKE ROGERS, Alabama
PAUL C. BROUN, Georgia
CANDICE S. MILLER, Michigan, *Vice Chair*
PATRICK MEEHAN, Pennsylvania
JEFF DUNCAN, South Carolina
TOM MARINO, Pennsylvania
JASON CHAFFETZ, Utah
STEVEN M. PALAZZO, Mississippi
LOU BARLETTA, Pennsylvania
RICHARD HUDSON, North Carolina
STEVE DAINES, Montana
SUSAN W. BROOKS, Indiana
SCOTT PERRY, Pennsylvania
MARK SANFORD, South Carolina
CURTIS CLAWSON, Florida

BENNIE G. THOMPSON, Mississippi
LORETTA SANCHEZ, California
SHEILA JACKSON LEE, Texas
YVETTE D. CLARKE, New York
BRIAN HIGGINS, New York
CEDRIC L. RICHMOND, Louisiana
WILLIAM R. KEATING, Massachusetts
RON BARBER, Arizona
DONALD M. PAYNE, JR., New Jersey
BETO O'ROURKE, Texas
FILEMON VELA, Texas
ERIC SWALWELL, California
VACANCY
VACANCY

BRENDAN P. SHIELDS, *Staff Director*
JOAN O'HARA, *Acting Chief Counsel*
MICHAEL S. TWINCHEK, *Chief Clerk*
I. LANIER AVANT, *Minority Staff Director*

(II)

CONTENTS

———

EBOLA IN THE HOMELAND: THE IMPORTANCE OF EFFECTIVE INTERNATIONAL, FEDERAL, STATE, AND LOCAL COORDINATION

Friday, October 10, 2014

U.S. HOUSE OF REPRESENTATIVES,
COMMITTEE ON HOMELAND SECURITY,
Dallas, TX.

The committee met, pursuant to call, at 12:10 p.m., in the In-Transit Lounge, D–31, Dallas-Fort Worth International Airport, 233 South International Drive, Dallas, Texas, Hon. Michael McCaul [Chairman of the committee] presiding.

Present: Representatives McCaul, Chaffetz, Sanford, Clawson, Thompson, Jackson Lee, Barber, O'Rourke, Vela, and Swalwell.

Also present: Representatives Farenthold, Marchant, Barton, Burgess, Veasey, and Johnson.

Chairman MCCAUL. The Committee on Homeland Security will come to order. The committee is meeting today to examine the coordinated Federal, State, and local response to the recent Ebola case right here in Dallas, Texas. First, I want to thank everybody, including the witnesses, for attending this hearing today, and I appreciate the efforts taken on behalf of all those involved to have this important field hearing.

This is an official Congressional hearing as opposed to a town hall, and as such, we must abide by certain rules of the committee and the House of Representatives. I would like to kindly remind our guests that demonstrations from the audience, including applause and verbal outbursts, as well as the use of signs or placards are a violation of the rules of the House of Representatives, and it is important that we respect the decorum and the rules of this committee. I have also been requested to state that photography and cameras are limited to accredited press only.

Before I recognize myself for an opening statement, I also ask unanimous consent that the gentlemen from Texas, Mr. Joe Barton, Mr. Michael Burgess, Mr. Kenny Marchant, Mr. Blake Farenthold, and Mr. Mark Veasey, and the gentlelady from Texas, Ms. Eddie Bernice Johnson, be permitted to sit on the dais and participate in today's hearing. Without objection, so ordered.

I will now recognize myself for an opening statement.

We are here today to discuss the threat to the United States homeland from the Ebola virus and what is being done to stop the spread of this terrible disease. This crisis is unfolding at an alarming pace. Thousands have died in Africa and thousands more have

(1)

been infected, including four selfless Americans working in Liberia who have been flown home for treatment.

Now the virus has begun to spread to other parts of the world, and the American people are rightfully concerned. They are concerned because the Ebola virus is an unseen threat, and it is only a plane flight away from our shores. We have witnessed that with the recent case here in Dallas, the first fatality from Ebola in the United States. But we must be sure to confront this crisis with the facts. Blind panic will not help us stop this disease from spreading, and fear-mongering will only make it harder to do so.

That is why we are here today, to ask the American people's questions and get answers from the experts. Americans are seeking assurance that our Federal, State, and local officials are doing everything in their power to keep this virus outside of the United States. Already there has been a vigorous international, Federal, State, and local response, and we hope to hear more today about exactly what has been done and what needs to be done going forward.

Two weeks ago, Thomas Eric Duncan traveled here from Liberia by way of Brussels and Dulles Airports. He fell ill and presented himself for treatment at Texas Health Presbyterian Hospital here in Dallas. Mr. Duncan's diagnosis set in motion an extensive public health operation involving Federal, State, and local officials to identify and assess any individuals with whom he may have had contact, a process called contact tracing. That contact tracing effort continues today, and our prayers are with everyone who is currently being monitored as part of this incident.

We are thankful that today there have been no additional cases of Ebola stemming from this case. Contact tracing is time-consuming and difficult, but it is one of the few ways to contain the disease. Containment also requires swift, coordinated action. In this committee's hearings and investigation on the Boston Marathon bombings, we heard testimony about the importance of the incident command system. The system is a vital tool for making sure first responders at all levels engage quickly and decisively rather than argue about who is in charge. The importance of such a response mechanism was highlighted in the 9/11 Commission Report, and it has since saved countless lives.

I was encouraged to learn officials here in Texas instituted the structure, and today State and Federal officials are co-located in the Dallas County Emergency Operations Center, enabling vital information sharing and coordination. To be clear, the situation here at home is far different than what is happening in West Africa. We have a strong public health infrastructure in place, particularly here in Texas, which enables us to work to contain this virus more effectively.

But Dallas is not the only area that we must be vigilant. We need to ensure that State and local responders Nation-wide are prepared to move quickly if the virus is detected anywhere else within our borders. Hospitals are recognizing this and have made nearly 190 inquiries with the CDC about cases they believe could be Ebola. Thankfully, testing was only warranted in about 24 of these cases, and only one case was confirmed as Ebola.

Public health and medical personnel must remain vigilant, ensure all hospital personnel are informed, follow protocols to identify the virus, and take appropriate quarantine measures. We must reinforce the importance of taking travel histories and sharing that information with all relevant personnel.

Protecting the homeland from the Ebola virus also requires us to put measures in place at our airports. I am pleased the President announced earlier this week additional entry screening efforts that are being launched. Beginning tomorrow, enhanced screening measures will be activated at JFK Airport, and soon after at Dulles, O'Hare, Newark, and Atlanta. These airports receive more than 94 percent of all travelers from Liberia, Sierra Leone, and Guinea. I look forward to hearing more about these enhanced screening efforts from our witnesses.

The Department of Homeland Security has been actively involved in this response, and I commend Secretary Johnson for his leadership. But we also must closely monitor the situation overseas and continue our global response efforts. I have spoken with the President's homeland security advisor, Lisa Monaco, numerous times to ensure our Government is doing all that is necessary. We recently discussed exit screening procedures that have been put in place in Liberia, Sierra Leone, and Guinea by CDC-trained personnel. In the past 2 months, the screening has stopped 77 travelers with Ebola-like symptoms or contact history from boarding airplanes out of a total of 36,000 individuals screened. Fortunately, none of those 77 have been diagnosed with Ebola.

While there have many positive aspects of this response, there have also been missteps. For instance, here in Dallas, Mr. Duncan's travel history was not communicated to all relevant medical personnel when he first sought treatment, which led to his release from the hospital and the potential that additional people were exposed to the virus. There were also problems removing hazardous biomedical waste from the apartment where Mr. Duncan's family was quarantined. The soiled materials remained in the home with the quarantined individuals for days after the Ebola diagnosis was confirmed.

We must learn from these missteps and ensure that proper procedures are established and followed should another case arise in the United States. Going forward, we must consider all policy options for stopping the spread of this horrific disease. I have heard many ideas directly from my fellow Texans, everything from stopping in-bound flights from specific countries to additional screenings at home and abroad. We hope our witnesses will discuss options that are being considered in the trade-offs that we have to confront.

We also have to ensure unnecessary Government red tape does not slow down the response. In fact, I know a reprogramming request was approved in the House seeking $750 million towards response efforts, and I would urge the Senate to follow the lead of the House and approve the Pentagon's request to transfer additional resources to this fight.

Now is not the time for politics. Congress has been loath to get anything done this session, and if there's ever been a time to come together and put pettiness aside, it is now. We must get this right and make sure that Federal protocols are put in place and communicated to our State and local partners when a situation this critical occurs. My hope today is that we do not focus on gotcha politics, but instead hear from our panel and focus on solutions. We are all in the same boat, and we need to work hard to make sure that our Nation is protected from this threat.

I want to thank the Ranking Member for being here today in my home State of Texas and showing his support for this shared goal. Before I turn it over to him, I would also like to commend our first responders, our medical personnel and public health officials, who have responded courageously to the case here in Dallas. Most importantly, our thoughts and prayers are with the victims and the families affected by this crisis. I look forward to hearing from the witnesses and hear from them what more can be done to keep Americans safe.

[The statement of Chairman McCaul follows:]

STATEMENT OF CHAIRMAN MICHAEL MCCAUL

OCTOBER 10, 2014

We are here today to discuss the threat to the U.S. homeland from the Ebola virus and what is being done to stop the spread of this terrible disease. The crisis is unfolding at an alarming pace. Thousands have died in Africa and thousands more have been infected, including 4 selfless Americans working in Liberia who have been flown home for treatment. Now the virus has begun to spread to other parts of the world, and the American people are rightfully concerned. They are concerned because the Ebola virus is an unseen threat, and it is only a plane-flight away from our shores. We've witnessed that with the recent case here in Dallas—the first fatality from Ebola in the United States.

But we must be sure to confront this crisis with the facts. Blind panic won't help us stop this disease from spreading, and fear-mongering will only make it harder to do so. That is why we are here today: To ask the American people's questions and get answers from our experts. Americans are seeking assurance that our Federal, State, and local officials are doing everything in their power to keep this virus out of the United States.

Already, there has been a vigorous international, Federal, State, and local response. We hope to hear more today about exactly what has been done—and what needs to be done going forward. Two weeks ago, Thomas Eric Duncan traveled here from Liberia by way of the Brussels and Dulles airports, fell ill, and presented himself for treatment at Texas Health Presbyterian Hospital here in Dallas. Mr. Duncan's diagnosis set in motion an extensive public health operation involving Federal, State, and local officials to identify and assess any individuals with whom he may have had contact, a process called "contact-tracing."

That contact-tracing effort continues today, and our prayers are with everyone who is currently being monitored as part of this incident. We are thankful that, to date, there have been no additional cases of Ebola stemming from this case. Contact-tracing is time-consuming and difficult, but it is one of the few ways to contain the disease. Containment also requires swift, coordinated action. In this committee's hearings and investigation on the Boston Marathon bombings, we heard testimony about the importance of the "incident command system."

The system is a vital tool for making sure first responders at all levels engage quickly and decisively, rather than argue over who is in charge. The importance of such a response mechanism was highlighted in the 9/11 Commission report, and it has since saved countless lives. I was encouraged to learn officials here in Texas instituted this structure. Today, State and Federal officials are co-located in the Dallas County Emergency Operations Center, enabling vital information sharing and coordination.

To be clear, the situation here at home is far different than what is happening in West Africa. We have a strong public health infrastructure in place, particularly here in Texas, which enables us to work to contain this virus more effectively. But Dallas is not the only area that must remain vigilant. We need to ensure that State and local responders Nation-wide are prepared to move quickly if the virus is detected anywhere else within our borders. Hospitals are recognizing this and have made nearly 190 inquiries with the CDC about cases they believed could be Ebola. Thankfully, testing was only warranted in about 24 of those cases, and only 1 case was confirmed as Ebola.

Public health and medical personnel must remain vigilant, ensure all hospital personnel are informed, follow protocols to identify this virus, and take appropriate quarantine measures. We must reinforce the importance of taking travel histories and sharing that information with all relevant personnel. Protecting the homeland from the Ebola virus also requires us to put measures in place out our airports. I am pleased the President announced earlier this week additional entry screening efforts are being launched. Beginning tomorrow, enhanced screening measures will be activated at JFK airport and soon after at Dulles, O'Hare, Newark, and Atlanta. These airports receive more than 94% of all travelers from Liberia, Sierra Leone, and Guinea. I look forward to hearing more about these enhanced screening efforts from our witnesses. The Department of Homeland Security has been actively involved in the response, and I commend Secretary Jeh Johnson for his leadership in bringing Federal resources to the fight.

We must also closely monitor the situation overseas and continue our global response efforts. I have spoken with the President's Homeland Security Advisor Lisa Monáco numerous times to ensure our Government is doing all that is necessary. We recently discussed exit screening procedures that have been put in place in Liberia, Sierra Leone, and Guinea by CDC-trained personnel. In the past 2 months, this screening has stopped 77 travelers with Ebola-like symptoms or contact history from boarding planes, out of a total of 36,000 individuals screened. None of those 77, that we are aware of, has been diagnosed with Ebola. While there have been many positive aspects of this response, there have also been missteps.

For instance, here in Dallas Mr. Duncan's travel history was not communicated to all relevant medical personnel when he first sought treatment, which led to his release from the hospital and the potential that additional people were exposed to the virus. There were also problems removing hazardous biomedical waste from the apartment where Mr. Duncan's family was quarantined. The soiled materials remained in the home with the quarantine individuals for days after the Ebola diagnosis was confirmed.

We must learn from these missteps, and ensure the proper procedures are established and followed should another case arise in the United States. Going forward, we must consider all policy options for stopping the spread of this horrific disease. I have heard many ideas directly from my fellow Texans—everything from stopping in-bound flights from specific countries to additional screenings at home and abroad. We hope our witnesses will discuss options that are being considered and the trade-offs we may have to confront.

We also have to ensure unnecessary Government red tape does not slow down the response. I urge the Senate to follow the lead of the House and approve the Pentagon's request to transfer additional resources to the fight. The Defense Department is seeking to move $750 million toward response efforts, and we should move swiftly to satisfy that request.

Now is not the time for politics. Congress has been loathe to get much done this session, and if there has ever been a time to come together and put pettiness aside, it is now. We must get this right and make sure that Federal protocols are put in place and communicated to our local and State leaders when a situation this critical occurs.

My hope today is we won't focus on gotcha politics, instead hearing from our panels and focusing on a solutions-based hearing. We are in the same boat. And we need to work hard to make sure that our Nation is protected from this threat. I want to thank the Ranking Member for being here in my home State of Texas in a show of support for this shared goal.

Before we begin, I also want to commend the first responders, medical personnel, and public health officials who have responded courageously to the case here in Dallas. Most importantly, our thoughts and prayers are with the victims and families affected by this crisis. I look forward to hearing from our distinguished panel of witnesses today on the recent response efforts and what more can be done to keep America safe.

Chairman MCCAUL. With that, the Chairman now recognizes the Ranking Member, Mr. Thompson.

Mr. THOMPSON. Good afternoon. I want to thank the Chairman for holding this timely hearing on our efforts, both domestic and international, to contain and prevent the spread of the Ebola virus. I also thank the witnesses for appearing here today, and I look forward to their testimony. Additionally, I want to thank Chair Biggins and the board of directors of the Dallas-Fort Worth Airport and executive staff for hosting the committee today.

I also want to extend my condolences to the family of Thomas Eric Duncan, the first person diagnosed with Ebola on American soil. We are not here to dehumanize Mr. Duncan, but unfortunately his diagnosis and the procedures that followed raise critical questions about our preparedness for highly infectious diseases, such Ebola, and how Federal, State, and local authorities coordinate in their aftermath.

As the Ranking Member of this committee, I often urge my colleagues not to use our positions of influence to promote fear in the public. Hence, I want to clarify that while it is proper to have serious concerns about the Ebola virus, it would be irresponsible for us to foster the narrative that an Ebola epidemic in the United States is imminent. Rather, this hearing provides us an opportunity to review our State, local, Federal, and global public health infrastructure, learn where there are inconsistencies and gaps, and lay the foundation for eliminating these disparities.

While the Ebola virus has caused the United States to institute new screening procedures at airports, it is incumbent upon us to work with our international partners to eradicate the virus at its origin in West Africa. The current Ebola outbreak is the deadliest outbreak on record. According to the Assistant Secretary General of the United Nations, it is also impairing National economies, wiping out livelihoods and basic services, and could undo years of efforts to stabilize West Africa. Eliminating this virus at its source is a sure-fire way to prevent more Ebola cases in the United States.

As citizens of the global community, it is our moral obligation to not only eradicate this virus that is devastating West Africa, but also ensure that these countries can continue to function and recover. The United States' response to the current Ebola outbreak will affect the ways it works to coordinate international responses to future disease outbreaks.

In this case, it seems as if the United States and the international community did not act aggressively soon enough. In March, the World Health Organization issued a notice of an Ebola outbreak in Guinea after the virus spread to Sierra Leone and Liberia. There was a lull in new cases in the spring, and as a result efforts waned. In June, Doctors Without Borders, a nongovernmental organization, declared the outbreak out of control. However, the World Health Organization and the international community did not improve on its efforts until August.

According to a chart that I have here, we had a lull until the spike started in August of this year. Mr. Chairman, I will submit for the record this chart.

Chairman MCCAUL. Without objection, so ordered.

[The information follows:]

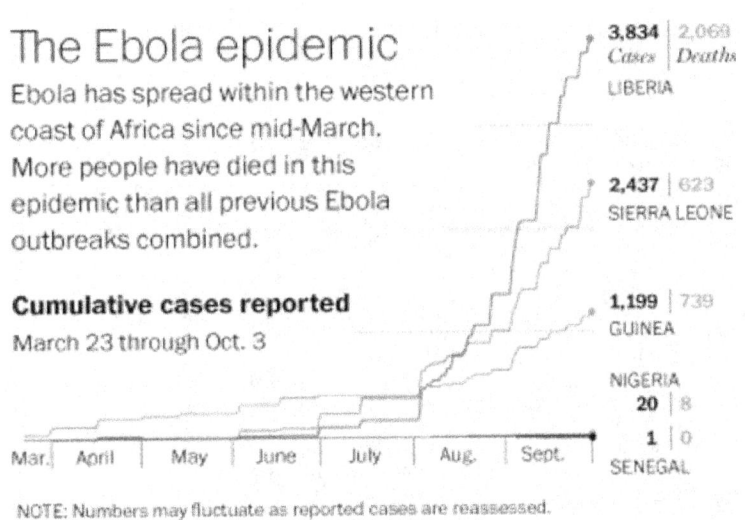

The Ebola epidemic

Ebola has spread within the western coast of Africa since mid-March. More people have died in this epidemic than all previous Ebola outbreaks combined.

Cumulative cases reported

March 23 through Oct. 3

3,834 | 2,069
Cases | Deaths
LIBERIA

2,437 | 623
SIERRA LEONE

1,199 | 739
GUINEA

NIGERIA
20 | 8

1 | 0
SENEGAL

Mar. | April | May | June | July | Aug. | Sept.

NOTE: Numbers may fluctuate as reported cases are reassessed.

Source: World Health Organization   THE WASHINGTON POST

Mr. THOMPSON. Thank you. Earlier I stated that an Ebola outbreak in the United States is not imminent. But what should be discussed post haste is the value of our public health infrastructure and the cost of maintaining it. Many times public health is used as a pawn for partisan bickering. However, Mr. Chairman, viruses such as Ebola, the flu, and EV–D68, which has affected over 500 children in the United States, do not know political parties.

Cuts to public health preparedness grants from the Department of Homeland Security, and Health and Human Services, the Centers for Disease Control, and the Office of the Surgeon General hit already struggling State and local health departments hard. As Members of Congress, we can use our platforms to restore grant funding and support the Federal cost of maintaining a public health infrastructure.

I hope that our discussion today can yield a step in this direction, and I also support the Chairman's comment that this disease does not see party or anything. It is an American problem that the world needs our best minds to address. I look forward, Mr. Chairman, to the testimony and witnesses and yield back the balance of my time.

[The statement of Ranking Member Thompson follows:]

STATEMENT OF RANKING MEMBER BENNIE G. THOMPSON

OCTOBER 10, 2014

I want to thank the Chairman for holding this timely hearing on our efforts—both domestic and international—to contain and prevent the spread of the Ebola virus. I also thank the witnesses for appearing today, and I look forward to their testimony. Additionally, I want to thank Chair Biggins and the board of directors of the Dallas Fort Worth Airport and the executive staff for hosting the committee today.

I also want to extend my condolences to the family of Thomas Eric Duncan, the first person diagnosed with Ebola on American soil. We are not here to dehumanize Mr. Duncan, but unfortunately his diagnosis and the procedures that followed raise critical questions about our preparedness for highly-infectious diseases such as Ebola and how Federal, State, and local authorities coordinate in their aftermath.

As Ranking Member of this committee, I often urge my colleagues not to use our positions of influence to promote fear in the public. Hence, I want to clarify that while it is proper to have serious concerns about the Ebola virus, it would be irresponsible for us to foster the narrative that an Ebola epidemic in the United States is imminent.

Rather, this hearing provides us the opportunity to review our State, local, Federal, and global public health infrastructure, learn where there are inconsistencies and gaps, and lay the foundation for eliminating these disparities. While the Ebola virus has caused the United States to institute new screening procedures at airports, it is incumbent upon us to work with our international partners to eradicate the virus at its origin in West Africa.

The current Ebola outbreak is the deadliest outbreak of record. According to the assistant secretary general of the United Nations, it is also impairing national economies, wiping out livelihoods and basic services, and could undo years of efforts to stabilize West Africa. Eliminating this virus at its source is a surefire way to prevent more Ebola cases in the United States.

As citizens of the global community, it is our moral obligation to not only eradicate this virus that is devastating West Africa, but also ensure that these countries can continue to function and recover. The United States' response to the current Ebola outbreak will affect the way it works to coordinate international responses to future disease outbreaks. In this case, it seems as if the United States and the international community did not act aggressively soon enough.

In March, the World Health Organization issued a notice of an Ebola outbreak in Guinea after the virus spread to Sierra Leone and Liberia. There was a lull in new cases in the spring, and as a result, efforts waned. In June, Doctors Without Borders, a non-Government organization, declared the outbreak out of control. However, the World Health Organization and the international community did not improve on its efforts until August. According to this chart from the *Washington Post,* the rate of new cases and fatalities appears to have grown exponentially during this time. We must do better, and I want to learn how the international community will be more engaged in the future.

Earlier, I stated that an Ebola outbreak in the United States is not imminent, but what should be discussed post haste is the value of our public health infrastructure and the cost of maintaining it. Many times, public health is used as a pawn for partisan bickering. However, viruses such as Ebola, the flu, and EV–D68 which has affected over 500 children in the United States do not know political parties.

Cuts to public health preparedness grants from the Departments of Homeland Security and Health and Human Services, the Centers for Disease Control, and the Office of the Surgeon General hit already struggling State and local health departments hard. As Members of Congress, we can use our platforms to restore grant funding and support the Federal costs of maintaining a public health infrastructure. I hope that our discussions today can yield a step in this direction.

Chairman MCCAUL. I thank the Ranking Member for his thoughtful comments and spirit of bipartisanship. Other Members are reminded that statements may be submitted for the record.

[The statement of Hon. Jackson Lee follows:]

STATEMENT OF HONORABLE SHEILA JACKSON LEE

OCTOBER 10, 2014

Good morning. I would like to begin by thanking Chairman McCaul and Ranking Member Thompson, for convening this hearing on "Ebola in the Homeland: The Importance of Effective International, Federal, State, and Local Coordination."

I would also like to thank all the witnesses testifying before us today:

- Dr. Toby Merlin, director of the Division of Preparedness and Emerging Infection Office for the National Center for Emerging and Zoonotic Infectious Diseases with the Center for Disease Control;
- Dr. Kathryin Brisfield, acting assistant secretary for health affairs and chief medical officer with the Department of Homeland Security;
- John P. Wagner, acting assistant commissioner, with the Office of Field Operations (OFO) with U.S. Customs and Border Protection;
- Dr. David L. Lakey, commissioner, Texas Department of State Health Services;

- Dr. Brett Giroir, executive vice president & CEO Texas A&M Health Science Center, who is also a professor in the College of Medicine at Texas A&M Health Science Center;
- Dr. Catherine L. Troisi, Ph.D., associate professor in the divisions of management, policy, and community health and epidimiology.
- The Hon. Clay Jenkins, judge, for Dallas County, TX.

Thank you all for being here and sharing your expertise and valuable experience with us as the Nation addresses the global Ebola crisis and the first U.S. patient, Mr. Thomas Eric Duncan, who became ill with Ebola after returning from West Africa and succumbed to the disease.

The topic of today's hearing clearly highlights the scope and responsibility of the House Committee on Homeland Security and the important role that the Homeland Security Department fulfills in protecting our Nation's people and securing our borders.

The World Health Organization reports that the numbers of deaths from Ebola is approaching 4,000. Medical experts are certain that this number is much higher than the deaths that have been reported.

Today, the goal of this committee, the Obama administration, and the governments around the world, both inside and outside of America, is to prevent Ebola from becoming the next AIDS.

As a senior Member of the House Committee on Homeland Security and the Ranking Member of the Subcommittee on Border Security, I am pleased that the Centers for Disease Control, the Department of Homeland Security's U.S. Customs and Border Protection Agency, and the United States Coast Guard are coordinating to establish a new level of screening for international air travelers during the global Ebola health crisis that is impacting the United States.

I understand this coordinated effort will add new screening protocols beginning Saturday, October 11, 2014 for passengers with flight itineraries originating in the countries of Guinea, Liberia, or Sierra Leone. I have requested that the George Bush Intercontinental Airport serving the Houston area be included among the airports where these protocols will be applied.

The Ebola virus cannot be ignored, it cannot be locked away and kept at bay, and it must be aggressively treated at its source—in Africa.

This is no time for hand-wringing or finger-pointing regarding this Ebola outbreak—this is the time for action. I commend this committee's leadership, President Obama; and the doctors and medical professionals who are bringing attention and resources to the forefront to stop this terrible disease.

I would offer that Members of this committee must renew our efforts to end sequestration. We cannot wage the fight that lies ahead without the full measure of resources that must be brought to contain and ultimately end this Ebola outbreak.

Ebola is not airborne.

It is only transmitted through body fluids when a person is symptomatic,—(i.e. has a fever from the disease and experiencing other symptoms.)

Incubation of the Ebola virus in victims can range from 2 to 21 days before signs of the illness emerge.

The Ebola virus is a single strain of RNA that is comprised of 7 genes that can attach to healthy red blood cells, invade the blood cell, and use the blood cell's environment to rapidly reproduce.

Typically a little over a week after exposure a patient may begin to exhibit symptoms, which include fever, chills, muscle pain, sore throat, weakness, and general discomfort.

The Ebola virus attacks immune cells in the bloodstream, which take the infection to the liver, spleen, and lymph nodes. Ebola then blocks the release of interferon, a protein made by immune cells to fight viruses.

At this stage of the infection, other tissues and organs can become compromised along with other cellular functions that disrupt vital organ function and autonomic processes that are carried out by cells.

Surviving Ebola requires the body to have time for the immune system to figure out how to fight the Ebola virus. Patients get time from receiving aggressive supportive care as early as possible in the Ebola infection process.

Supportive care begins with proper identification of symptoms and signs of the disease causing stress or distress to organs or body functions and using the appropriate symptom management treatments.

Active treatment to stave off the effects of the disease can include:

1. ibuprofen to address fevers;
2. transfusion of blood to deal with bleeding, moderate to severe pallor or signs of emergency circulatory shock;
3. pain reduction; and

4. difficulty in respiration and dehydration.

Providing supportive care as early as possible to stabilize the Ebola victim and allow the patient's immune system time to learn how to fight the disease is the most important factor for successful recovery.

There are several experimental treatments that have been used in patients, but it is too early to say whether these medicines have made a difference in their recoveries.

The disease is not just a threat to the patient; it also poses a significant threat to first-line responders that provide critical health care to Ebola patients.

Doctors Without Borders have developed a very detailed and care process that health care workers around the world must follow without deviation to make sure that they are protected, while providing care to Ebola patients.

The posture of the United States must be one of vigilance, and for this reason, I recently wrote to President Obama to thank him for his leadership, both globally and Nationally, in addressing the threats posed by the largest Ebola outbreak in history.

I mentioned earlier, I also requested that George Bush Intercontinental Airport be included on the list of airports to receive the enhanced Ebola screening protocols for those passengers whose flight itineraries indicate that the air travel originated in the countries of Guinea, Liberia, or Sierra Leone.

The George Bush Intercontinental Airport serves the Houston area and is a major originating and connecting hub for international air travelers. From January to August 2014, there were 99,452 West African passengers traveling into and out of the George Bush Intercontinental Airport with a total of 1,856,421 international travelers.

In 2013 nearly 40 million passengers traveled through the George Bush Intercontinental Airport of which 8.9 million were international travelers.

George Bush Intercontinental Airport ranks as the 9th largest airport in the United States for flight operations and ranks as one of our Nation's busiest airports.

I requested that George Bush Intercontinental Airport be added to the list of airports receiving new layers of entry screening.

I look forward to the testimony of today's witnesses and what they believe we are doing to be helpful to them in their work and where we can do better in supporting their efforts to stop the spread of Ebola.

Once again, I would like to thank you Chairman McCaul and Ranking Member Thompson for convening this hearing. I yield back the balance of my time.

Thank you.

Chairman MCCAUL. We have a very distinguished panel of experts here today. First, Dr. Toby Merlin is the director of the Division of Preparedness and Emerging Infections at the National Center for Emerging and Zoonotic Infectious Disease at the U.S. Centers for Disease Control and Prevention, CDC. In this role, he is responsible for the CDC's Laboratory Response Network, infectious disease emergency response coordination, and emerging infections epidemiology, and laboratory capacity programs. Thank you for being here, sir.

Next, Dr. Kathryn Brinsfield serves as the acting assistant secretary of health affairs and chief medical officer for the Department of Homeland Security's Office of Health Affairs. She began her service with DHS in July 2008. She previously served as associate chief medical officer and director of the Division of Workforce, Health, and Medical Support within OHA. Prior to serving as acting assistant secretary, she served on a detail to the National security staff as the director of medical preparedness policy. Thank you so much for being here.

Last, Mr. John Wagner. I want to thank you for the tour you gave me earlier of this facility and how you would deal with potential Ebola victims coming through this airport. Mr. Wagner became acting assistant commissioner, Office of Field Operations, for Customs and Border Protection in April 2014. In his current position, he oversees nearly 28,000 employees with more than 22,000 CBP

Officers and CBP Ag Specialists that protect our borders. An annual operating budget of $3.2 billion provides for operations at over 329 ports of entry and programs that support National security, immigration, customs, and commercial trade related to the missions.

The full written statements will appear in the record. The Chairman now recognizes Dr. Merlin for 5 minutes.

STATEMENT OF TOBY MERLIN, M.D., DIRECTOR, DIVISION OF PREPAREDNESS AND EMERGING INFECTION, NATIONAL CENTER FOR EMERGING AND ZOONOTIC INFECTIOUS DISEASES, CENTERS FOR DISEASE CONTROL AND PREVENTION, U.S. DEPARTMENT OF HEALTH AND HUMAN SERVICES

Dr. MERLIN. Thank you, and good afternoon, Chairman McCaul, Members of the committee, and members of the Texas delegation. I appreciate the opportunity to be here today to discuss the current epidemic of Ebola in West Africa, as well as the work CDC is doing to manage the global consequences of this epidemic. I have been particularly involved with colleagues here in Dallas addressing the first U.S.-diagnosed Ebola case, and like you, our hearts go out to the family and friends of Mr. Duncan. As CDC Director Dr. Frieden noted, "Mr. Duncan puts a real face on the epidemic for all Americans."

The Ebola epidemic in Guinea, Liberia, and Sierra Leone is ferocious and continues to spread exponentially. The current outbreak is the first that has been recognized in West Africa, and the biggest and most complex Ebola epidemic ever documented. As of last week, the epidemic surge passed 7,900 cumulative reported cases and nearly 3,800 documented deaths, though we believe the numbers could be 2 or 3 times higher.

Fortunately, the United States and others in the global community are intensifying our response in order to bring this critical situation under control. From the time the situation in West Africa escalated from an outbreak to an epidemic, we have anticipated that a traveler might arrive in the United States with the disease. The imported case of Ebola in Dallas required the CDC and the Nation's public health system to implement rapid response protocols that have been developed in anticipation of such an event.

Within hours of confirming that the patient had Ebola, CDC had a team of 10 people on the ground in Dallas to assist the capable teams from the Texas State Health Department and local authorities. We have worked side-by-side with State and local health officials to prevent infections of others. Together, we assessed all 114 individuals who might have possibly had contact with the patient. We narrowed down the contacts to 10 who may have been around the patient when he was infectious, and 30 others with whom possible infection could not be ruled out. These individuals are being tracked and will be tracked for 21 days for any signs of symptoms, and they will quickly be isolated if symptoms develop.

We are also working to identify and learn lessons from the initial patient encounter and other events that complicated our response, and to apply them in any other responses. We are confident that our public health and health care systems can prevent an Ebola outbreak here, and that the authorities and investments provided by Congress have put us in a strong position to protect Americans.

To make sure the United States is prepared as the epidemic in West Africa has intensified, CDC has done the following. No. 1, it has instituted layers of protection starting in affected countries where our staff work intensively on airport exit screening. No. 2, we have provided guidance for airline personnel and for agents from DHS on how to identify sick passengers and how to manage them.

No. 3, along with partners in DHS and State and local health agencies, we have continually assessed and improved approaches to in-bound passenger screening and management. As the President announced on October 6, CDC is working with DHS to intensify the screening at United States' airports. This is something my colleagues from DHS will be discussing this morning.

We have worked with American hospitals to reinforce and strengthen infection controls. Fifth, with State health departments, we have intensified training and outreach to build awareness. Six, we have expanded lab capacity across the United States to test for Ebola. Seven, we have developed response protocols for the evaluation, isolation, and investigation of symptomatic individuals. We have extensively consulted to support evaluation, and when indicated, testing of suspected cases.

We remain confident that Ebola is not a significant public health threat to the United States. It is not transmitted easily, and it does not spread from people who are not ill. It is possible that another infected traveler might arrive in the United States. Should this occur, we are confident that our public health and health care systems can prevent the kind of significant transmission of Ebola that would lead to an outbreak here in the United States.

It is important to remember that the only way to protect Americans, though, is to end this Ebola epidemic and to continue our intensive focus on West Africa, and there implement proven public health interventions. Working with our partners, we have been able to stop every previous Ebola outbreak, and we are determined to stop this one. It will take meticulous work, and we cannot take shortcuts.

Thank you again for the opportunity to appear before you today and for making CDC's work on this epidemic and other health threats possible. Thank you, Mr. Chairman.

[The prepared statement of Dr. Merlin follows:]

PREPARED STATEMENT OF TOBY MERLIN

OCTOBER 10, 2014

Good afternoon Chairman McCaul, Members of the committee, and members of the Texas Delegation. Thank you for the opportunity to testify before you today and for your on-going support for the Centers for Disease Control and Prevention's (CDC) work in global health. I am Dr. Toby Merlin, director of CDC's Division of Preparedness and Emerging Infections. I appreciate the opportunity to be here today to discuss the epidemic of Ebola in West Africa, as well as the work the CDC is doing to manage the global consequences of this epidemic in the wake of the first diagnosed case here in the United States 2 weeks ago, which ultimately and tragically, has become the first death from Ebola in the United States.

From the time the situation in West Africa escalated from an outbreak to an epidemic, we have anticipated that a traveler could arrive in the United States with the disease. We have been preparing for this possibility by working closely with our

State and local partners and with clinicians and health care facilities so that any imported case could be quickly contained. This occurrence underscores the need to carefully follow the protocols that have been developed, to work closely across levels of government, and to continue our urgent effort to address the epidemic in West Africa, which remains the biggest risk to the United States.

As we work to learn from the recent case in Dallas and continue the public health response there, we remain confident that Ebola is not a significant public health threat to the United States. It is not transmitted easily, and it does not spread from people who are not ill, and cultural norms that contribute to the spread of the disease in Africa—such as burial customs—are not a factor in the United States. We know how to stop Ebola with strict infection control practices which are already in wide-spread use in American hospitals, and the United States is leading the international effort to stop it at the source in Africa. CDC is committing significant resources both on the ground in West Africa and through our Emergency Operations Center here at home.

We have been constantly monitoring our response in the United States, and will continue to do so. The CDC and the U.S. Customs & Border Protection (CBP) in the Department of Homeland Security (DHS) announced this week that we will begin new layers of entry screening at five U.S. airports that receive over 94 percent of travelers from the Ebola-affected nations of Guinea, Liberia, and Sierra Leone. New York's JFK International Airport will begin the new screening October 11. In the 12 months ending July 2014, JFK received nearly half of all travelers from those three West African nations. The enhanced entry screening will also be implemented at Washington-Dulles, Newark, Chicago-O'Hare, and Atlanta international airports.

This is a whole-of-Government response, with agencies across the United States Government committing human and financial resources. Across HHS, CDC is actively partnering with the Office of Global Affairs, the Office of the Assistant Secretary for Preparedness and Response, the National Institutes of Health, and the Food and Drug Administration to coordinate and respond to this epidemic. Also, CDC has embedded technical staff in the USAID-led DART team in West Africa. Additionally, staff, logistical support, and resources from the Department of Defense (DoD) are already being deployed to rapidly scale up our efforts to include constructing Ebola treatment units and training health care workers. We are working closely with our international partners to scale up the response to the levels needed to stop this epidemic.

Ebola is a severe, often fatal, viral hemorrhagic fever. The first Ebola virus was detected in 1976 in what is now the Democratic Republic of Congo. Since then, outbreaks have appeared sporadically. The current epidemic in Guinea, Liberia, and Sierra Leone is the first time an outbreak has been recognized in West Africa, the first-ever Ebola epidemic, and the biggest and most complex Ebola challenge the world has ever faced. We have seen cases imported into Nigeria and Senegal from the initially-affected areas and we have also seen in Nigeria and Senegal that proven practices such as contact tracing can contribute to managing Ebola and preventing a small number of cases from growing into a larger outbreak.

Ebola has symptoms similar to many other illnesses, including fever, chills, weakness and body aches. Gastrointestinal symptoms such as vomiting and diarrhea are common and profound, with fluid losses on average of 5–7 liters in 24 hours over a 5-day period. These fluid losses can result in life-threatening electrolyte losses. In approximately half of cases there is hemorrhage—serious internal and external bleeding. There are two things that are very important to understand about how Ebola spreads. First, the current evidence suggests human-to-human transmission of Ebola only happens from people who are symptomatic—not from people who have been exposed to, but are not ill with the disease. Second, everything we have seen in our decades of experience with Ebola indicates that Ebola is not spread by casual contact; Ebola is spread through direct contact with bodily fluids of someone who is sick with, or has died from Ebola, or exposure to objects such as needles that have been contaminated. While the illness has an average 8–10 day incubation period (though it may be as short as 2 days and as long as 21 days), we recommend monitoring for fever and signs of symptoms for the full 21 days. Again, we do not believe people are contagious during that incubation period, when they have no symptoms. Evidence does not suggest Ebola is spread through the air. Catching Ebola is the result of exposure to bodily fluids, which we are seeing occur in West Africa, for example, in hospitals in weaker health care systems and in some African burial practices. Getting Ebola requires exposure to bodily fluids of someone who is ill from—or has died from—Ebola.

The earliest recorded cases in the current epidemic were reported in March of this year. Following an initial response that seemed to slow the early outbreak for a time, cases flared again due to weak systems of health care and public health and because of challenges health workers faced in dealing with communities where critical disease-control measures were in conflict with cultural norms. As of last week, the epidemic surpassed 7,900 cumulative reported cases, including nearly 3,800 documented deaths, though we believe these numbers may be substantially under-reported. The effort to control the epidemic in some places is complicated by fear of the disease and distrust of outsiders. Security is tenuous and unstable, especially in remote isolated rural areas. There have been instances where public health teams could not do their jobs because of security concerns.

Many of the health systems in the affected countries in West Africa are weak or have collapsed entirely, and do not reach into rural areas. Health care workers may be too few in number or may not reliably be present at facilities, and those facilities may have limited capacity. Health care workers are at greater risk of Ebola due to conditions they are working in and we must work to reduce that risk. Poor infection control in routine health care, along with local traditions such as public funerals and cultural mourning customs including preparing bodies of the deceased for burial, make efforts to contain the illness more difficult. Furthermore, the porous land borders among countries and remoteness of many villages have greatly complicated control efforts. The secondary effects now include the collapse of the underlying health care systems resulting for example, in an inability to treat malaria, diarrheal disease, or to safely deliver a child, as well as non-health impacts such as economic and political instability and increased isolation in these areas of Africa. These impacts are intensifying, and not only signal a growing humanitarian crisis, but also have direct impacts on our ability to respond to the Ebola epidemic itself.

Fortunately, we know what we must do. In order to stop an Ebola outbreak, we must focus on three core activities: Find active cases, respond appropriately, and prevent future cases. The use of real-time diagnostics is extremely important to identify new cases. We must support the strengthening of health systems and assist in training health care providers. Once active cases have been identified, we must support quality patient care in treatment centers, prevent further transmission through proper infection control practices, and protect health care workers. Epidemiologists must identify contacts of infected patients and follow up with them every day for 21 days, initiating testing and isolation if symptoms emerge. And, we must intensify our use of health communication tools to disseminate messages about effective prevention and risk reduction. These messages include recommendations to report suspected cases, to avoid close contact with sick people or the deceased, and to promote safe burial practices. In Africa, another message is to avoid bush meat and contact with bats, since "spillover events," or transmission from animals to people, in Africa have been documented through these sources.

Many challenges remain. While we do know how to stop Ebola through meticulous case finding, isolation, and contact tracing, there is currently no cure or vaccine shown to be safe or effective for Ebola. We are working to strengthen the global response, which requires close collaboration with the World Health Organization (WHO) and additional assistance from our international partners. At CDC, we activated our Emergency Operations Center to respond to the initial outbreak, and are surging our response. As of last week, CDC has over 139 staff in West Africa, and over 1,000 staff in total have provided logistics, staffing, communication, analytics, management, and other support functions. CDC will continue to work with our partners across the United States Government and elsewhere to focus on key strategies of response:

- *Effective incident management.*—CDC is supporting countries to establish National and sub-National Emergency Operations Centers (EOCs) by providing technical assistance and standard operating procedures and embedding staff with expertise in emergency operations. All three West African countries at the center of the epidemic have now named and empowered an Incident Manager to lead efforts.
- *Isolation and treatment facilities.*—It is imperative that we ramp up our efforts to provide adequate space to treat the number of people afflicted with this virus.
- *Safe burial practices.*—Addressing local cultural norms on burial practices is one of the keys to stopping this epidemic. CDC is providing technical assistance for safe burials.
- *Infection control throughout the health care system.*—Good infection control will greatly reduce the spread of Ebola and help control future outbreaks. CDC has a lead role in infection control training for health care workers and safe patient triage throughout the health care system, communities, and households.
- *Communications.*—CDC will continue to work on building the public's trust in health and Government institutions by effectively communicating facts about the disease and how to contain it, particularly targeting communities that have presented challenges to date.

The public health response to Ebola rests on the same proven public health approaches that we employ for other outbreaks, and many of our experts are working in the affected countries to rapidly apply these approaches and build local capacity. These include strong surveillance and epidemiology, using real-time data to improve rapid response; case-finding and tracing of the contacts of Ebola patients to identify those with symptoms and monitor their status; and strong laboratory networks that allow rapid diagnosis.

The resources provided for the period of the Continuing Resolution will support our response and allow us to ramp up efforts to contain the spread of this virus. More than half of the funds are expected to directly support staff, travel, security and related expenses. A portion of the funds will be provided to the affected area to assist with basic public health infrastructure, such as laboratory and surveillance capacity, and improvements in outbreak management and infection control. Should other outbreaks occur in this region, authorities will have the experience and capacity to respond without a massive external influx of aid, due to this investment. The remaining funds will be used for other aspects of strengthening the public health response such as laboratory supplies/equipment, and other urgent needs to enable a rapid and flexible response to an unprecedented global epidemic. CDC is working to identify our potential resource needs for the rest of the fiscal year, and possibly further, as we deal with this evolving situation. CDC will continue to coordinate activities directly with critical Federal partners, including the United States Agency for International Development (USAID), DoD, DHS, and non-Governmental organizations. Over the past few weeks, we have seen progress, as the DoD has begun deploying assets to the area and laying the ground work to construct 17 Ebola treatment facilities, train local workers to staff the facilities, and move supplies into the area. In addition, USAID is working closely with non-Governmental organizations to scale up efforts in all areas of the response. Currently, there are over 50 burial teams in all 15 counties of Liberia for the management of safe human remains. More than 70 organizations are providing Ebola education and awareness in Liberia, Guinea, and Sierra Leone. Organizations are also working to increase infection control practices in all health facilities to ensure functionality of the health care system. We continue to work with national governments, WHO, and USAID to provide for interim measures such as isolation in community settings with proper protections, and improvements to ensure the safe burial of those who have died from the virus.

Though the most effective step we can take to protect the United States is to stop the epidemic where it is occurring, we are also taking strong steps to protect Americans here at home. The imported case of Ebola in Dallas, diagnosed on September 30 in a traveler from Liberia, required CDC and the Nation's public health system to implement rapid response protocols that have been developed in anticipation of such an event. Within hours of confirming that the patient had Ebola, CDC had a team of 10 people on the ground in Dallas to assist the capable teams from the Texas State health department and local authorities. We have worked side-by-side with State and local officials to prevent infection of others. Together, we assessed all 114 individuals who might possibly have had contact with the patient. We narrowed down the contacts to 10 who may have been around the patient when he was infectious and 38 others with whom infection cannot be ruled out. These individuals will be tracked for 21 days for any signs of symptoms, and they will quickly be isolated if symptoms develop. We are also working to identify and learn lessons from the initial patient encounter and other events that complicated our response, and to apply them in any other responses. We are confident that our public health and health care systems can prevent an Ebola outbreak here, and that the authorities and investments provided by the Congress have put us in a strong position to protect Americans. To make sure the United States is prepared, as the epidemic in West Africa has intensified, CDC has done the following:

- Instituted layers of protection, starting in affected countries where our staff work intensively on airport exit screening, such as temperature scanning for outbound passengers.
- Provided guidance for airline personnel and for DHS Customs and Border Protection Officers on how to identify sick passengers and how to manage them. Though it was one of many false alarms, the recent incident with an in-bound passenger to Newark, New Jersey shows how CDC's quarantine station at the airport worked with airline, DHS, airport, EMS, and hospital personnel to assess and manage a sick passenger, and to protect other passengers and the public.
- Developed guidance for monitoring and movement of people with possible exposures.

- Along with partners in DHS and State and local health agencies, continually assessed and improved approaches to in-bound passenger screening and management, and as the President announced on October 6, CDC is working with DHS to enhance screening measures at United States airports.
- Worked with American hospitals to reinforce and strengthen infection controls, and CDC has provided checklists and instructions to all health care facilities to assess patients for travel history. We have also worked with State and local health departments to ensure that these practices are being followed.
- With State health departments, intensified training and outreach to build awareness since the Dallas case.
- Through the Laboratory Response Network (LRN), expanded lab capacity across the United States—in addition to CDC's own world-class laboratories, 14 LRN labs now have capacity for testing, ensuring that we have access to labs for timely assessment—and surge capacity in case it is needed.
- Developed response protocols for the evaluation, isolation, and investigation of any incoming individuals with relevant symptoms.
- Extensively consulted to support evaluation and, when indicated, tested suspect cases. With heightened alert, we are receiving hundreds of inquiries for help in ruling out Ebola in travelers—a sign of how seriously airlines, border agents, and health care system workers are taking this situation. So far just over a dozen of these hundreds of suspect cases have required testing, and only one (the Dallas patient) has been positive.

Our top priority at CDC is to protect Americans from threats. We work 24/7 to do that. In the case of Ebola, we are doing that in many different ways here at home, but we also need to retain our focus on stopping the outbreak at its source, in Africa.

Working with our partners, we have been able to stop every prior Ebola outbreak, and we will stop this one. It will take meticulous work and we cannot take short cuts. It's like fighting a forest fire: Leave behind one burning ember, one case undetected, and the epidemic could re-ignite. For example, in response to the case in Nigeria, 10 CDC staff and 40 top Nigerian epidemiologists rapidly deployed, identified, and followed 1,000 contacts for 21 days. Even with these resources, one case was missed, which resulted in a new cluster of cases in Port Harcourt. However, due to the meticulous work done in Nigeria, no new cases have been identified, and the outbreak appears to have been extinguished there.

Ending this epidemic will take time and continued, intensive effort. Before this outbreak began, we had proposed, in the fiscal year 2015 President's budget, an increase of $45 million to strengthen lab networks that can rapidly diagnose Ebola and other threats, emergency operations centers that can swing into action at a moment's notice, and trained disease detectives who can find an emerging threat and stop it quickly. Building these capabilities around the globe is key to preventing this type of event elsewhere and ensuring countries are prepared to deal with the consequences of outbreaks in other countries. We must do more, and do it quickly, to strengthen global health security around the world, because we are all connected. Diseases can be unpredictable—such as H1N1 coming from Mexico, MERS emerging from the Middle East, or Ebola in West Africa, where it had never been recognized before—which is why we have to be prepared globally for anything nature can create that could threaten our global health security.

Investments in strengthening health systems in West Africa have been very challenging due to the low capacity of the systems. However, all of the donor partners agree that adequately strengthening the public health infrastructure in West Africa could allow such outbreaks to be detected earlier and contained. This Ebola epidemic shows that any vulnerability could have wide-spread impact if not stopped at the source.

In February, the United States Government joined with partner governments, WHO and other multilateral organizations, and non-Governmental actors to launch the Global Health Security Agenda (GHSA). Over the next 5 years, the United States has committed to working with over 40 partner countries (with a combined population of at least 4 billion people) to improve their ability to prevent, detect, and effectively respond to infectious disease threats—whether naturally-occurring or caused by accidental or intentional release of pathogens. As part of this Agenda, the President's fiscal year 2015 budget includes $45 million for CDC to accelerate progress in detection, prevention, and response, and we appreciate your support for this investment. We are working to evaluate the needs to strengthen the Ebola-affected nations and neighboring ones most at risk, and are asking that GHSA partners make specific commitments to establish capacity in West African countries in 2 or 3 years to prevent, detect, and rapidly respond to infectious disease threats. The economic cost of large public health emergencies can be tremendous—the 2003

Severe Acute Respiratory Syndrome epidemic, known as SARS, disrupted travel, trade, and the workplace and cost to the Asia-Pacific region alone $40 billion. Resources provided for the Global Health Security Agenda can improve detection, prevention, and response and can potentially reduce some of the direct and indirect costs of infectious diseases.

Improving these capabilities for each nation improves health security for all nations. Stopping outbreaks where they occur is the most effective and least expensive way to protect people's health. While this tragic epidemic reminds us that there is still much to be done, we know that sustained commitment and the application of the best evidence and practices will lead us to a safer, healthier world. With a focused effort, and increased vigilance at home, we can stop this epidemic, protect Americans, and leave behind a strong system in West Africa and elsewhere to prevent Ebola and other health threats in the future.

Thank you again for the opportunity to appear before you today. I appreciate your attention to this terrible epidemic and I look forward to answering your questions.

Chairman McCAUL. Thank you, Dr. Merlin.

The Chairman recognizes Dr. Brinsfield for her testimony.

STATEMENT OF KATHRYN BRINSFIELD, M.D., M.P.H., F.A.C.E.P, ACTING ASSISTANT SECRETARY AND CHIEF MEDICAL OFFICER, OFFICE OF HEALTH AFFAIRS, U.S. DEPARTMENT OF HOMELAND SECURITY

Dr. BRINSFIELD. Chairman McCaul, Ranking Member Thompson, distinguished Members, thank you for inviting me to speak with you today. I appreciate the opportunity to testify on the Department of Homeland Security's role in the Federal Government's Ebola response. I am also honored to testify alongside my colleagues from the Centers for Disease Control and Prevention and U.S. Customs and Border Protection. I also want to thank the Texas State and local officials who will be testifying later. DHS works closely with the State of Texas on a number of important issues, and we appreciate their hard work, coordination, and collaboration.

As you know, DHS is responsible for securing our Nation's borders and safeguarding the American public from communicable disease that threaten to traverse our borders, including Ebola. The DHS Office of Health Affairs is at the intersection of homeland security and public health with a mission to advise, promote, integrate, and enable a safe and secure workforce in the Nation in pursuit of National health security. OHA achieves this by enhancing the health and wellness of the DHS workforce, and by protecting the Nation from the health impacts of events, including diseases of public health significance.

In my role as acting chief medical officer for the Department, I provide medical and health expertise to DHS components and senior leadership. In this capacity, I am helping to coordinate with components and provide them with medical advice regarding the Department's efforts in preparing for and responding to Ebola.

As my CDC colleague has noted, the 2014 Ebola epidemic is the largest Ebola in history, and it has had devastating impacts in multiple West African countries, the hardest-hit being Liberia, Sierra Leone, and Guinea. On September 30, 2014, CDC confirmed the first travel-associated case of Ebola in the United States. The patient had traveled from Liberia to Dallas, Texas, connecting through the Brussels airport in Belgium and Dulles in Virginia. Sadly, he has since passed away.

The patient did not have symptoms when he left Liberia, nor when he entered the United States, but developed them approximately 5 days after his arrival. The public concern surrounding this event and possible future public exposure to Ebola from international travelers is understandable, although it is important to remember that the CDC has stated that the risk of an Ebola outbreak in the United States is very low.

The President has been focused every day on the Government's response, and has stated to his senior health, homeland security, and National security advisors that the epidemic in West Africa is a top National security priority. DHS takes this issue very seriously and has been closely monitoring the Ebola virus since its outbreak in April.

We are actively engaged in the Ebola response working with our Federal and international partners to develop multiple mechanisms to allow screening at different stages of transit to minimize the potential spread of Ebola outside of West Africa. We are closely monitoring this situation, actively engaged with our State and local partners and adjusting our processes as needed.

DHS has executed a number of measures to minimize the risk of individuals with Ebola from entering the United States, and we take a layered approach to ensure there are varying points at which an ill individual could be identified so that there is no single point of failure. To this end, DHS is also focused on protecting those traveling by air and taking steps to ensure that passengers with communicable diseases like Ebola are screened, identified, isolated, and quickly and safely referred to medical personnel. We have been working with the CDC to implement an additional layer of screening for travelers entering the United States, which is scheduled to begin this weekend.

These additional screening protocols are just some of the many actions the Federal Government has taken in our layered approach to help ensure the risk of Ebola in the United States remains minimal. Assistant Commissioner Wagner will go into more detail regarding the specific measures CBP is taking, but I would like to highlight some other key actions we at DHS have taken to date and will continue to take.

CBP and the Transportation Security Administration have posted messages from the CDC at select airport locations that provide awareness on how to prevent the spread of infectious disease, typical symptoms of Ebola, and instructions to call a doctor if the traveler becomes ill. TSA is engaging with industry partners and domestic and foreign air carriers to provide awareness on the current outbreak, and has issued an information circular to air carriers reinforcing the CDC's message on Ebola and providing guidance on identifying potential passengers with Ebola.

OHA through our National Biosurveillance Integration Center is continuing to monitor the outbreak and is producing tailored Ebola products. These reports are disseminated to more than 15,000 Federal, State, and local public health and law enforcement officials. The U.S. Coast Guard is monitoring vessels known to be inbound from Ebola-affected countries, and is providing information to the captain of the port, district, and CDC representatives.

DHS is also committed to ensuring that our own employees have up-to-date information. We have provided our personnel with health advisories on the current outbreak, including impacted regions, symptoms of the virus, and mode of transmission, and operational procedures and precautions.

The Department of Homeland Security has worked closely with its interagency partners to develop a layered approach to Ebola response. DHS is always assessing the measures we have in place and will consider additional actions moving forward if appropriate to protect the American people. I look forward to working with you to address any concerns or questions.

[The joint prepared statement of Dr. Brinsfield and Mr. Wagner follows:]

JOINT PREPARED STATEMENT OF KATHRYN BRINSFIELD AND JOHN WAGNER

OCTOBER 10, 2014

Chairman McCaul, Ranking Member Thompson, distinguished Members of the committee, and the Texas Delegation, we appreciate the opportunity to submit this statement on the U.S. Customs and Border Protection's (CBP) and the Office of Health Affairs' (OHA) roles in the Federal Government's Ebola response.

The 2014 Ebola epidemic is the largest in history with devastating impacts in multiple West African countries—the hardest-hit being Liberia, Sierra Leone, and Guinea. In the midst of this public health event, it is important to remember that the Centers for Disease Control and Prevention (CDC) has stated that the risk of a widespread Ebola outbreak in the United States is very low. OHA and CBP, as part of the Department of Homeland Security's (DHS) overall strategy, are engaged on a daily basis with DHS interagency partners to prepare for and respond to Ebola and other potential threats to public health.

As you know, DHS is responsible for securing our Nation's borders and assisting the Department of Health and Human Services (HHS) in safeguarding the American public from communicable diseases that threaten to traverse our borders. In doing so, DHS is committed to ensuring that our responses to the Ebola epidemic are conducted consistent with established civil rights and civil liberties protections. OHA is at the intersection of homeland security and public health, better known as health security. OHA provides medical and health expertise to DHS components and senior leadership, and is helping to coordinate with components and provide them with medical advice regarding the Department's efforts in preparing for and responding to Ebola. In today's remarks, we will provide an overview of the Department's efforts to protect the American people from Ebola, and CBP's specific efforts within ports of entry to identify and respond to travelers who may pose a threat to public health.

As the Nation's unified border security agency, CBP is responsible for securing our Nation's borders while facilitating the flow of legitimate international travel and trade that is so vital to our Nation's economy. Within this broad responsibility, CBP's priority mission remains to prevent terrorists and terrorist weapons from entering the United States. CBP also plays an important role in limiting the introduction, transmission, and spread of serious communicable diseases from foreign countries.

The President has been focused every day on this response and has stated to his senior health, homeland security, and National security advisors that the epidemic in West Africa is a top National security priority, and that we will continue to do everything necessary to address it. Because of the steps we have taken, the President reiterated that he is confident that the chances of an outbreak in the United States are extraordinarily low.

SCREENING AND OBSERVATION PROTOCOLS

CBP and the CDC have closely coordinated to develop policies, procedures, and protocols to identify travelers to the United States who may have a communicable disease, responding in a manner that minimizes risk to the public. These pre-existing procedures—applied in the land, sea, and air environments—have been utilized collaboratively by both agencies on a number of occasions with positive results.

As a standard part of every inspection, CBP Officers observe all passengers as they arrive in the United States for overt signs of illness, and question travelers, as appropriate, at all U.S. ports of entry. CBP Officers are trained in illness recognition by the CDC. Officers look for overt signs of illness and can obtain additional information from the travelers during the inspection interview. If a traveler is identified with overt signs of a communicable disease of public health significance, the traveler is isolated from the traveling public and referred to CDC's Regional Quarantine Officers or local public health for medical evaluation.

It is important to note that the CDC has worked closely with affected countries, and CBP has provided support and assistance, to ensure that all out-bound travelers from the areas affected by the West Africa Ebola outbreak are screened for Ebola symptoms before departure. CDC provides "Do Not Board" recommendations to CBP and the Transportation Security Administration (TSA) regarding individuals who may be infected with a highly contagious disease, present a threat to public health, and should be prevented from traveling via commercial aircraft. TSA is performing vetting of all airline passengers coming to, departing from or flying within the United States to identify matches to the "Do Not Board" list and flag matched individuals' records in the Secure Flight system to prevent the issuance of a boarding pass. TSA is also supporting CDC requirements to identify all passenger reservations on flights where it has been determined that one or more passengers present an Ebola risk, such as when passengers have traveled from the affected African areas and have exhibited Ebola symptoms.

ADDITIONAL EBOLA SCREENING MEASURES

Although we have recently seen the first cases of Ebola virus in the United States, the CDC believes that the U.S. clinical and public health systems will work effectively to prevent the spread of the Ebola virus. DHS has executed a number of measures to minimize the risk of those sick with Ebola entering the United States, and we take a layered approach to ensure there are varying points at which an ill individual could be identified. To this end, DHS is also focused on protecting the air traveling public and taking steps to ensure that travelers with communicable diseases like Ebola are identified, isolated, and quickly and safely referred to medical personnel.

On October 21, DHS announced travel restrictions in the form of additional screening and protective measures at our ports of entry for travelers from the three Ebola-affected countries in West Africa. As of October 22, all passengers arriving in the United States whose travel originated in Liberia, Sierra Leone, or Guinea are required to fly into one of five airports including New York John F. Kennedy; Washington Dulles; Newark; Chicago O'Hare; and Atlanta International Airport. DHS is working closely with the airlines to implement these restrictions with minimal travel disruption.

At these five airports, all travelers from the affected countries undergo enhanced screening measures consisting of targeted questions and a temperature check, through the use of non-contact thermal thermometers, seeking to determine whether the passengers are experiencing symptoms or may have been exposed to Ebola. Detailed contact information is also collected in the event the CDC needs to contact them in the future. If there is reason to believe a passenger has been exposed to Ebola, either through the questionnaire, temperature check, or overt symptoms, CBP refers the passenger to CDC for further evaluation. The CDC has surged staff to these airports to support this mission requirement.

In addition to these measures, CBP Officers are asking all passengers traveling on a passport from Liberia, Sierra Leone, and Guinea, regardless of where they traveled from, whether they have been in one of the three countries in the prior 21 days. If the traveler has been in one of the three countries in the prior 21 days, he or she will be referred for additional screening and, if necessary, CDC or other medical personnel in the area will be contacted pursuant to existing protocols.

The U.S. Coast Guard is also monitoring vessels known to be in-bound from Ebola-affected countries, and is providing information to the Captain of the Port, District, and CDC representatives.

The CDC maintains Federal jurisdiction to determine whether to isolate or quarantine potentially-infected arrivals. DHS personnel may be called upon to support the enforcement of the CDC's determinations, and we stand ready to help.

INFORMATION SHARING AND TRAINING

DHS has prioritized sharing information and raising awareness as important elements in combating the spread of Ebola, and CBP has a unique opportunity to deliver critical information to targeted travelers from the affected countries in ports of entry. Secretary Johnson recently directed CBP to distribute health advisories to all travelers arriving in the United States from the Ebola-affected countries of Liberia, Sierra Leone, and Guinea. These advisories provide the traveler with information on Ebola, health signs to look for, and information for their doctor should they need to seek medical attention in the future.

CBP and TSA have posted messages from the CDC at select airport locations that provide awareness on how to prevent the spread of infectious disease, typical symptoms of Ebola, and instructions to call a doctor if the traveler becomes ill in the future.

We also share information with our non-Governmental and State and local partners. TSA is engaging with industry partners and domestic and foreign air carriers to provide awareness on the current outbreak, and has issued an Information Circular to air carriers reinforcing the CDC's message on Ebola and providing guidance on identifying potential travelers with Ebola.

OHA, through the National Biosurveillance Integration Center, is continuing to monitor the outbreak to coordinate information in response to the event. These reports on biological events are disseminated to more than 15,000 Federal, State, and local users, many of whom work in the public health sector or support 78 fusion centers across the Nation, helping to ensure that the most up-to-date information is available.

DHS is committed to ensuring that our own employees have up-to-date and accurate information. We have provided our own personnel with background information on the current outbreak, information on the regions of importance; symptoms of the virus and mode of transmission; and operational procedures and precautions for processing travelers showing signs of illness. CBP field personnel will be kept up to date on National, regional, and location-specific information on Ebola preparedness and response measures through regular field musters. CBP has provided guidance to the field on baggage inspection for international travelers from impacted countries, proper procedures for inspection and handling of prohibited meat products, and proper safeguarding and disposal of garbage from all in-bound international flights.

CBP Officers receive the CDC's public health training, which teaches officers to identify symptoms and characteristics of ill travelers. CBP also provides operational training and guidance to front-line personnel on how to respond to travelers with potential illness, including referring individuals who display signs of illness to CDC quarantine officers for secondary screening, the use of personal protective equipment (which is available for employees at these airports along with instructions for use), as well as training on assisting CDC with implementation of its isolation and quarantine protocols. CBP Officers are trained to employ universal precautions, an infection control approach developed by the CDC, when they encounter individuals with overt symptoms of illness or contaminated items in examinations of baggage and cargo. Universal precautions assume that every direct contact with body fluids is infectious and requires exposed employees to respond accordingly. TSA also ensures that its employees are adequately trained and, where appropriate, are provided personal protective equipment. The health and safety of DHS employees is also our priority as we carry out this critical mission.

CONCLUSION

The Department of Homeland Security has worked closely with its interagency partners to develop a layered approach to identifying ill travelers and protecting the air traveling public. DHS is always assessing the measures we have in place and continues to look at any additional actions that can be taken to ensure the safety of the American people. We look forward to working with you to address this problem collaboratively. We will continue to closely monitor the Ebola outbreak, and will evaluate additional measures as needed.

We thank you for your time and interest in this important issue. We look forward to answering your questions.

Chairman McCAUL. Thank you, Dr. Brinsfield.

Mr. Wagner, you are recognized for 5 minutes.

STATEMENT OF JOHN WAGNER, ACTING ASSISTANT COMMISIONER, OFFICE OF FIELD OPERATIONS, U.S. CUSTOMS AND BORDER PROTECTION, U.S. DEPARTMENT OF HOMELAND SECURITY

Mr. WAGNER. Thank you, Chairman McCaul, Ranking Member Thompson, and distinguished Members of the committee for the opportunity to discuss the efforts of U.S. Customs and Border Protection in deterring the spread of Ebola by means of international travel.

Each day CBP processes over 1 million people into the United States. About 280,000 of them enter at our international airports each day. CBP is responsible for securing our Nation's borders while facilitating the flow of legitimate trade and travel that is so vital to our Nation's economy.

Within this broad responsibility, our priority mission remains to prevent terrorists and terrorist weapons from entering the United States. However, we also play an important role in limiting the introduction, transmission, and spread of serious communicable diseases from foreign countries. We have had this role for over 100 years, and as travel and threats change, CBP has changed as well.

In coordination with CDC, we have modern protocols in place for well over a decade that have guided response to a variety of a significant health threats over recent years. CBP Officers at all ports of entry assess each traveler for overt signs of illness. In response to the recent Ebola virus outbreak in West Africa, CBP in close collaboration with the DHS Office of Health Affairs and the Centers for Disease Control and Prevention is working to ensure that front-line officers are provided the information, training, and equipment needed to identify and respond to international travelers who may pose a threat to public health.

All CBP Officers are provided guidance and training on identifying and addressing travelers with any potential illness, including communicable diseases, such as the Ebola virus. CBP Officer training includes CDC public health training, which teach officers to identify through visual observation and questioning the overt symptoms and characteristics of ill travelers.

CBP also provides operational training and guidance on how to respond to travelers with potential illness, including referring individuals who display signs of illness to CDC quarantine officers for secondary screening, as well as training on assisting CDC with implementation of its isolation and quarantine protocols. Additionally, CBP provides web-based training for its front-line personnel, covering key elements of CBP's blood-borne pathogens, exposure control plan, protections from exposure, use of personal protective equipment, and other preventive measures and procedures to follow in a potential exposure incident.

We are committed to ensuring our field personnel have the most accurate, updated information regarding the Ebola virus. Since this outbreak began, CBP field personnel have been provided a steady stream of guidance starting with initial information on the current outbreak at the beginning of April this year with numerous and regular updates since then. We have provided field personnel information on the regions of importance, the symptoms of the virus, and modes of transmission, and operational procedures and precautions for processing passengers showing signs of illness.

We will continue to provide our officers National, regional, and location-specific——

Voice. Is your mic on, sir?

Mr. Wagner. Yes.

Voice. Can you lift your mic up?

Mr. WAGNER. Absolutely. Sorry.

VOICE. Thank you.

Mr. WAGNER. We will continue to provide our officers National, regional, and location-specific information on Ebola preparedness and response measures through field musters. We have also provided guidance to the field on baggage inspection for travelers from impacted countries, proper procedures for inspection and handling of prohibited meat products, and proper safeguard against disposal of garbage from all in-bound international flights.

Information sharing is critical, and CBP continues to engage with health and medical authorities at the National, State, and local level. Since January 2011, CDC's Division of Global Migration and Quarantine has stationed a liaison officer at the CBP National Targeting Center to provide subject-matter expertise and facilitate requests for information between the two organizations. CBP has also been actively engaged with the air carrier industry and other Federal partners regarding Ebola preparedness and potential response operations.

Now, in response to the current outbreak, CBP identifies travelers whose travel originated in or transited through Guinea, Liberia, and Sierra Leone. Starting October 1, CBP began providing a CDC Ebola travel health alert notice to travelers entering the United States from these affected countries. This information notice provides the traveler information and instructions should he or she have a concern of possible infection.

In addition to visually screening all passengers for overt signs of illness, starting October 11, CBP and CDC will begin enhanced screening of travelers from the three affected countries entering JFK Airport given that a significant number of travelers from the affected countries enter at JFK. In coordination with CDC, these targeted travelers will be asked to complete a CDC questionnaire, provide contact information, and have their temperature checked. Based on these enhanced screening efforts, CDC Quarantine Officers will make a public health assessment.

These enhanced efforts will roll out next week at Dulles, O'Hare, Atlanta, and Newark. Combined approximately 94 percent of all travelers from the affected countries entering the United States come through these five airports. CBP will continue to screen for overt signs of illness on all passengers, and will also provide Ebola tear sheets to travelers at all other locations who come in from these affected countries.

While CBP Officers receive training in illness recognition and response, if they identify an individual believed to be ill, we will separate the traveler from the public and contact the local CDC Quarantine Officer along with local public health authorities to help with a further medical assessment.

CBP will continue to monitor the Ebola outbreak, provide timely information and guidance to our field personnel, and work closely with DHS and our interagency partners to develop or adopt measures as needed to deter the spread of Ebola in the United States. So thank you for the opportunity to testify today, and thank you for the attention you are giving to this very important issue. I am happy to questions.

Chairman MCCAUL. Thank you. The Chairman recognizes himself for questions. You know, like any threat overseas, we would rather eliminate that threat before it can get into the United States, and this threat is no exception.

I commend the efforts overseas in Africa to contain and control this. Part of that effort are flights into western Africa with health care officials to help stop the spread of this viral disease. But many of my constituents and many Americans are asking the question, why are we not banning all flights from West Africa into the United States. So, Dr. Merlin, I want to give you an opportunity to answer that question. Why should we not ban all flights from West Africa into the United States?

Dr. MERLIN. Mr. Chairman, I appreciate the opportunity to speak to that because I know it is a concern of many people. The disease outbreak in Liberia, Guinea, and Sierra Leone is now at a point where we may be able to stop it if we focus our efforts and our resources on stopping it. In order to stop it, we need uninhibited transit into and out of the country so that we can bring the resources there to bear that are needed to stop it, as well as to keep the countries from collapsing.

If we do not do that, the disease will grow exponentially. Our projections are there could be from 400,000 to 1.4 million cases by the end of the year if we do not do anything. There is no way in that circumstance to prevent disease from spilling from those countries into neighboring countries and then out into the rest of the world. So our opportunity now is to get the disease at its source. What we want is to not do things that may give the appearance currently of protecting us, but actually put us at greater risk later on by allowing the disease to grow there.

Chairman MCCAUL. I appreciate that. Dr. Brinsfield.

Dr. BRINSFIELD. So, sir, we work closely with our partners in CDC. We work through an interagency process with this. DHS is prepared to take any steps necessary, but want to make sure that we defer the public health expertise in this issue to CDC.

Chairman MCCAUL. Dr. Merlin, you said that this is not a significant health threat to the United States, I believe, in your testimony. Dr. Brinsfield, you said the risk is very low. I wanted to see if you could elaborate on that and explain how this deadly, wicked virus is actually transmitted.

Dr. MERLIN. Thank you, Mr. Chairman. As you say, the virus is a horrible virus because it causes horrible disease. In people who are infected, it has a high mortality rate. But we know a lot about this virus, and we know from 40 years' experience how to stop outbreaks of this virus. The virus is acquired by people by direct contact from infected individuals who are symptomatic. They do not get the disease from contact with people who are asymptomatic. It is often contacted by people caring for an individual who is infectious and sick.

After acquisition, there is an incubation period where the person who has acquired the virus is not him or herself symptomatic. That incubation period ranges usually about 8 to 11 days. It can be shorter. It can be longer. But then when the person develops symptoms, and only when the person develops symptoms, is the person capable of spreading the disease to other individuals.

Chairman McCAUL. Dr. Brinsfield.

Dr. BRINSFIELD. I would agree, sir. I would also point out as the USAID director has stated, this is a disease that preys on poor public health and poor public infrastructure. We have excellent public health and public infrastructure in this country.

Chairman McCAUL. As I understand, it is bodily fluid contact rather than influenza, which would be airborne.

Dr. BRINSFIELD. That is correct, sir. That is our current knowledge.

Chairman McCAUL. I think a lot of people want to know at what point are we going to have a treatment, or a cure, or vaccine for this disease. Where are we? What is the latest on that?

Dr. MERLIN. Mr. Chairman, I will provide a brief overview. There are a number of investigational countermeasures that are being explored for either vaccinating to prevent Ebola or drugs or biologics that can be used to treat Ebola. The time course when those would be available on a size and scale to treat large populations is fairly prolonged. The clinical trials with a vaccine will not take place until early next year.

Chairman McCAUL. I would hope that the clinical trials would be expedited in this case.

Dr. MERLIN. They are being expedited as quickly as possible. I should, you know, also say that this work is not work that CDC itself does, but it is work that is done by NIH and BARDA. They can provide more details on it. The point I wanted to make is that these countermeasures, although they may be available on an investigational new drug basis to treat occasional cases in the United States and occasional cases in Africa now, they are not a method that we can use now to attack the outbreak, the epidemic in Africa. What we need to use now is the standard public health methods of isolating infectious people so they do not spread the disease to other individuals, and safe burials of people because their bodies are infectious and they need to be handled appropriately.

Chairman McCAUL. Lastly, Dr. Brinsfield, in the Clinton and Bush administrations, they had a senior biodefense advisor in the White House to coordinate Federal, State, and local efforts. That position was eliminated in the current administration. Do you know why that was eliminated, and who is responsible now for coordinating at the Federal, State, and local level?

Dr. BRINSFIELD. I think, sir, that we have a very robust interagency process. We have meeting regularly on this issue and this particular disease for months. We believe very strongly that the different and varied expertises available are all necessary to come to the table and make educated decisions.

Chairman McCAUL. I thank you. The Chairman now recognizes the Ranking Member.

Mr. THOMPSON. Thank you very much, Mr. Chairman. When I left the Jackson, Mississippi airport this morning, the news talked about this hearing. A number of people saw me, and they wanted to know: Is it safe, what do I have to have? So needless to say, it is on the minds of a lot of people in this country.

To that extent, Dr. Merlin, I think it is important that to the extent that we can sing off the same page of music as we push information out, the better off we are. Can you provide this committee with how that process works from a public health standpoint and notification to State and local partners around the country?

Dr. MERLIN. Mr. Thompson, I will tell you how the process works for identification of cases. Is that what you would like me——

Mr. THOMPSON. That is fine.

Dr. MERLIN. Okay. We have worked with our Federal partners and our State and local partners to distribute information to health departments, to health department personnel, as well as to hospitals and physicians on the signs and symptoms of Ebola, the travel history that is there for Ebola, and how to detect Ebola infections.

We on our website have provided a checklist for facilities. We have provided guidance for facilities on how to do this. We have provided guidance on how facilities and physicians should handle an individual who they think is suspected of Ebola and how they can place them in isolation immediately so that they do not infect others, and we have provided testing for Ebola diagnostics around the country. We offer 24/7 consultative services through the CDC for people who have questions about how to handle a suspected case. Am I addressing your——

Mr. THOMPSON. That is it, but I want to go to a simpler reference. Some people are saying, well, we had two people to come and get treated from West Africa who lived, and Mr. Duncan came and died. The public is trying to say, what happened? I think we have to somehow provide a level of confidence to the public that the difference is still part of the system. Can you help me, if not other Members of the committee, with a response for that?

Dr. MERLIN. Yes, I will. Ebola is a horrible disease, as many people have said. The virus infects many parts of the body and interferes with the functions of many parts of the body. It is in the gastrointestinal tract. It is in the heart. It is in the liver. It is in the skin. People develop profound diarrhea and profound nausea and vomiting. The outcome of untreated Ebola cases is a mortality of from 50 to 90 percent, depending on a number of factors, including the age of the person.

We have limited experience with treating Ebola with our developed medical system, and the outcomes are dependent on a number of factors. A lot have to do with preexisting illness in the patient, how quickly after onset of symptoms the patient receives therapy. So I wish we had the assumption that every person who comes down with Ebola who gets Western-style medicine would survive, but I do not think that is the case.

Mr. THOMPSON. Thank you. Mr. Wagner, you talked a little bit about this enhanced screening that we will start implementing. I want to give you a scenario, and I want you to help me with an answer. If someone buys a ticket in West Africa to Brussels and then buys another ticket from Brussels to the United States, will that enhanced targeting pick that person up, or is that still a vulnerability we need to address?

Mr. WAGNER. It could be a vulnerability depending on how the airline has provided us with the information. If it is a continuous ticket, we will absolutely see it. If it is multiple tickets, we may not. In that case, we would use our officer that interviews the person when they arrive in the United States, and they flip through the passport booklet to look for stamps to see where they have been.

Everyone goes through a series of questions just about purpose and intent of travel, so we may ask the person, you know, how long were they were in Brussels and what were they doing there. When the answer is, well, I was transiting there, we could ask from where. So from our questioning we should be able to determine where that travel originated. Also on the customs declaration, we ask people what countries they are traveling from and where they have been to. So there are a few different ways we would find that out.

Mr. THOMPSON. Thank you. Yield back, Mr. Chairman.

Chairman McCAUL. The Chairman now recognizes Mr. Chaffetz.

Mr. CHAFFETZ. Thank you. I thank the Chairman and the Ranking Member for holding this hearing on such an important topic. Mr. Wagner, I would like to start with you by first recognizing the people in Customs and Border Protection, the men and women who do a very difficult job, very demanding job day in and day out. We appreciate, love them, and care for them. They have our thoughts and prayers as they have a very tough duty, and then to add this on top of it is obviously——

I want to talk about the legal authority and what you are able to do. Being sick is not illegal, but if they are coming here and they are from a suspected region, a suspected country, and they do appear to be sick, and they do not want to be detained, if they do want to, what can you do and not do?

Mr. WAGNER. So if they are not a U.S. citizen or permanent resident, some of our immigration authorities allow us to declare someone inadmissible to the United States if they have certain communicable diseases. Other than that, you know, we do screening of all the people just for overt signs of illness in general, and then we can work with CDC on some of their authorities to detain and quarantine or isolate sick travelers that would have it.

Mr. CHAFFETZ. So if somebody is appearing to be sick and they are a United States citizen, but they have been in, say, Liberia, what can you do or not do at that point?

Mr. WAGNER. We would closely with CDC then and use some of their authorities to get——

Mr. CHAFFETZ. But what is that authority? I am just wondering how far you can take this, what you can do or not do.

Dr. MERLIN. I am not a person at CDC who is familiar with all of CDC's quarantine authorities. But CDC has statutory authority to quarantine people who are suspected of having infectious diseases that are a risk to the public health. We can do that through any of our quarantine stations, and we can work with CBP so that——

Mr. CHAFFETZ. So can you help me understand what the standard is? Is it going to be if you have traveled to those countries, if you have the sniffles? What is the standard?

Dr. MERLIN. No. I will have to get back to you on the exact details of that. It certainly is more than you say. It would have to be, you know, a reasonable suspicion that the person could cause harm and infect other individuals by entering the country, and the person needs to be placed in isolation.

Mr. CHAFFETZ. So if they are a United States citizen, not a United States citizen, does that come into play?

Dr. MERLIN. Not from our perspective. If they are a threat to the public health and they need to be in isolation, we will exercise our legal authority.

Mr. CHAFFETZ. So what determines the threat to public health?

Dr. MERLIN. That is an area that I am afraid I do not know, and I——

Mr. CHAFFETZ. But if you do not know, how are the men and women are supposed to, you know, be screening somebody in 2 minutes and they have got a line of 12 people behind them, they are pressured. If you, Dr. Merlin, do not know that, how are Mr. Wagner's people supposed to figure it out?

Dr. MERLIN. I wish I knew all of these things in detail, but we actually a division of people who focus on quarantine and migration.

Mr. CHAFFETZ. I guess my concern is we are starting this new process. You have articulated the need, and if you do not know it, how is Mr. Wagner's—by the thousands we have to train and teach people how to identify this and then pull the right people out of a line. So when will you have that?

Dr. MERLIN. Well, fortunately Mr. Wagner works with people at CDC who do know this.

Mr. CHAFFETZ. Okay. So, Mr. Wagner, what is the answer to this question?

Mr. WAGNER. So, we will identify the travelers with the overt symptoms. We then contact CDC for the medical professionals to make that determination as to what meets that standard and what the follow-up care is going to be.

Mr. CHAFFETZ. Is that only going to happen at the five ports? What if it happens in Salt Lake City, and they are coming out?

Mr. WAGNER. We do that at all our locations now.

Mr. CHAFFETZ. There is a CDC representative at every port of entry.

Mr. WAGNER. No, we have 20 locations where they are located at. But we have contact information for them at all of our ports of entry, and if we encounter a traveler that has overt signs of illness, we will contact CDC and coordinate with them.

Mr. CHAFFETZ. So you are going to hold those people until CDC shows up?

Mr. WAGNER. We potentially could depending on the nature of what it is. That——

Mr. CHAFFETZ. So if they have got a high fever, they are from Liberia, and they are showing up, they are trying to walk through the port at Nogales, what are you going to do?

Mr. WAGNER. I would think we would stop them and call CDC and contact them until we could get some medical guidance about what they wanted to do with that person. But at the end of the day, that is going to be the medical professionals that make those determinations, not CBP.

Mr. CHAFFETZ. Mr. Chairman, I guess the encouragement here is somehow we need to CDC to come up with some really, good teachable standards so that the people in Mr. Wagner's Customs and Border Protection actually know what to look for and then what to actually do. If we do not have that information, we are going to make this job impossible. So, again, I thank you for holding this hearing, and I yield back.

Chairman MCCAUL. Yes, and for clarification, though, Dr. Merlin, you said there is a division devoted to this legally.

Dr. MERLIN. Yes. There is an entire division at CDC that is devoted to quarantine and migration.

Chairman MCCAUL. Do they coordinate with CBP?

Dr. MERLIN. They coordinate with CBP. What I would do if the question were asked of me by someone in the CBP section, I would immediately get in touch with someone who knows the answer to this question.

Chairman MCCAUL. The Chairman now recognizes the gentlelady from Texas, Ms. Jackson Lee.

Ms. JACKSON LEE. Mr. Chairman and Ranking Member, let me thank you very much for this vital hearing and the expression of the concern of the Members of the United States Congress. I thank my colleagues for their presence. I particularly, again, as I note thank my Chairman and Ranking Member, and I thank several Members that are from this region. I thank them so very much for their engagement and participation in this on-going challenge.

I know that we will see some of our local officials on the second panel, but I want to acknowledge them now and appreciate all the work that the county and all of the first responders have done in this community. We need to express our appreciation to them. Certainly I thank all of you for your presence here today and the very valiant work that you have done.

Ten days ago I was at Bush Intercontinental Airport, and I raised the red flag, not the historical flag, as I was able to be escorted by Customs and Border Protection to look at the very fine men and women who work there. I visited the containment unit by CDC. We were told on the day that I visited that my CDC team was here in Dallas. I saw the equipment that was there. I went down to the sub-basement to look at the amount of equipment. When I say "equipment," I think it is the Tyvek suits that are there to ensure that both CDC and others have it. So I think that it is important for the American public to know that stocked in many of the airports is this kind of equipment, but I raised the red flag to ensure that there was this kind of screening.

Publicly today I am going to make a request and think there was an error made by not designating Bush Intercontinental Airport as one of the sites to have this enhanced screening. I have made a request to the President, and to the Secretary, and to the Centers for Disease Control, and I hope that this will be responded to. Again, this is a red flag. This is not hysteria. It is based upon the travel that comes into Bush Intercontinental Airport.

Let me also say that it is not West Africa, and all of us must be restrained in how we define it. It is particular countries such as Guinea, Liberia at this time, and Sierra Leone. In fact, I offer this headline that says "Sierra Leone Leader Pleads for Ebola Aid," which means that we are interrelated.

The President has done a remarkable job, and I want to thank him for the 130 civilians, the ETU units. These are the containment units that have been set up. The 50 site burial teams, and of course, $350 million and another $700 million, I believe, that I hope that the Congress and all of us will convince the Congress to support. I especially want to thank the men and women of the United States military, particularly from Fort Bliss and Fort Hood that are now on their way or soon to be on their way.

But let me raise this question. I took the time to talk to some of our medical professionals at Baylor and the Harris Health System, which is our county health system. They indicated that—let me stop for a moment and join my colleague by expressing my sympathy to Mr. Duncan's family, and, again, pray for them as they mourn his passing, and take a moment to do that.

But I want to just relate to you where I think infrastructure and practical implementation may be two distinct things. We have the greatest health system in the world, but are we practically prepared? I do not think that we are practically prepared, and that is why we are having this oversight hearing.

If you have any indication of an Ebola patient, I would think with not any condemnation, you clear out any hospital. Patients are not going to come. So the question is: Do we need to—Dr. Merlin, I just need a yes or no—do we need to put contagion units together?

I hear from my health professionals in this flu season that hospitals are saying when persons have those similar symptoms and they are just an average citizen, that they are getting pushback on the ambulances to bring people with those kinds of symptoms. You have already indicated it is vomiting. It is quite different, but they are alike, similar. Do you think it would be appropriate to have those kinds of units? I know you are seeing them in the hospitals. Do you think they need to be separately placed?

Dr. MERLIN. I understand the question, and, no, I think that all facilities need to be able to care for people who present to those facilities for care. We cannot rely on individuals to present to selected facilities. All facilities need——

Ms. JACKSON LEE. Let me go on——

Dr. MERLIN. Sure.

Ms. JACKSON LEE [continuing]. To the next question, and I want to ask one to Mr. Wagner before my runs out. This question goes to the two medical persons. I am told that in a survey by nurses that they are telling me across the country, 80 percent are saying that the hospitals have not communicated to them any policy regarding potential admission of patients infected by Ebola. Eighty-five percent say their hospital has not provided education on Ebola with the ability for the nurses to interact. I am going to ask to put this into record. One-third say their hospital has insufficient supplies of eye protection, face shields, et cetera.

Chairman MCCAUL. Without objection.

[The information follows:]

EVEN AFTER DALLAS, HOSPITALS STILL LAGGING IN PREPARATION FOR U.S. EBOLA
PATIENTS

National Nurses United Press Release, 10/6/14

*85% say their hospital has not provided proper training, education in response
to possible Ebola infection*

News of the first confirmed patient in the U.S. infected with the Ebola virus still
has not led to effective communication with registered nurses who would be among
the first to respond and interact with patients possibly infected, according to survey
responses from at least 1,400 registered nurses across the U.S.

National Nurses United is stepping up the call on U.S. hospitals to immediately
upgrade emergency preparations for Ebola in this country.

"Nurses know that what is critical now in the face of this deadly disease is to
spread readiness, not fear. It is Ebola today, but other infectious diseases are not
far away. All hospitals need to take steps now to protect patients, frontline caregivers, and public safety," said Bonnie Castillo, RN, who directs NNU's disaster re-
lief program, Registered Nurse Response Network.

Several weeks ago, National Nurses United began surveying registered nurses
across the U.S. about emergency preparedness. Most of the nurses are telling NNU
that they remain unaware of proper preparation for the Ebola virus.

As of Monday morning, about 1,400 RNs at more than 250 hospitals in 31 states
have responded to the NNU national survey. Notably, the number of RNs responding has more than tripled since the news of the Dallas case—and yet the over-
whelming number of RNs voicing concern over lack of preparedness at their hospitals has showed virtually no improvement.

Current findings show:
- Nearly 80 percent say their hospital has not communicated to them any policy
  regarding potential admission of patients infected by Ebola.
- 85 percent say their hospital has not provided education on Ebola with the ability for the nurses to interact and ask questions.
- One-third say their hospital has insufficient supplies of eye protection (face
  shields or side shields with goggles) and fluid resistant/impermeable gowns.
- Nearly 40 percent say their hospital does not have plans to equip isolation
  rooms with plastic covered mattresses and pillows and discard all linens after
  use, fewer than 10 percent said they were aware their hospital does have such
  a plan in place.

NNU is calling for all U.S. hospitals to immediately implement a full emergency
preparedness plan for Ebola, or other disease outbreaks. That includes:
- Full training of hospital personnel, along with proper protocols and training ma-
  terials for responding to outbreaks, with the ability for nurses to interact and
  ask questions.
- Adequate supplies of Hazmat suits and other personal protective equipment.
- Properly equipped isolation rooms to assure patient, visitor, and staff safety.
- Proper procedures for disposal of medical waste and linens after use.

"Handing out a piece of paper with a link to the Centers for Disease Control, or
telling nurses just to look at the CDC website—as we have heard some hospitals
are doing—is not preparedness. Hospitals can and must do better, and we should
have uniform national standards and readiness," Castillo said.

The Dallas case, where the infected patient was sent home after arriving at the
hospital, hardly provides any reassurance, said NNU.

Media reports have indicated that the Dallas patient's exposure was not properly
communicated to hospital staff. But, Castillo added, it's not just a failure to commu-
nicate, but also a reminder that hospitals should not just rely on automated protocols with computerized scripts for interacting with patients.

"It's time to move from the electronic computer plan to a national healthcare action plan," said Castillo. "We have the expert nurses and physicians, we have to
train and drill with the whole team, from triage to treatment to waste disposal."

"As we have been saying for many months, electronic health records systems can,
and do, fail. That's why we must continue to rely on the professional, clinical judgment and expertise of registered nurses and physicians to interact with patients, as
well as uniform systems throughout the U.S. that are essential for responding to
pandemics, or potential pandemics, like Ebola," Castillo said.

Finally, Castillo said criminalizing the patient in Dallas or elsewhere is "exactly
the wrong approach and will do nothing to stop Ebola or any other pandemic."

NNU is also calling for significant increases in provision of aid, financial, personnel, and protective equipment, from the U.S., other governments, and private

corporate interests to the nations in West Africa directly affected to contain and stop the spread of Ebola.

Ms. JACKSON LEE. Your answer to how you are going to get all hospitals prepared, and, Mr. Wagner, your answer on airports that are not in this scheme of several airports, what are your men and women doing, and where do they take these patients if they find they are infected? Dr. Merlin, you can answer about this survey by nurses who say that they are actually not prepared.

Dr. MERLIN. That is concerning, and we will reach out to our State and local health departments and medical and hospital associations to see that those things are addressed. Nurses need to feel that they practice in a safe environment and that they can deal with patients who are potentially infectious, whether it is something like Ebola or something as simple as influenza. They need to have the needed personal protective equipment, and we will follow up on that.

Ms. JACKSON LEE. Mr. Wagner, if he is able to answer the question. What are you doing in airports that are not in this five-member——

Chairman MCCAUL. If the gentleman would answer the question. We do need to keep to the 5-minute rule. We have 16 Members of Congress. Go ahead and answer.

Mr. WAGNER. Okay. So any location outside of the five, what we will do is we will identify their travel as originating from one of those areas, and we will provide them with an information notice about the symptoms of Ebola and where to go for help and assistance if they start to develop these symptoms and where they can go get additional information.

Chairman MCCAUL. Thank you. The Chairman now recognizes Mr. Sanford.

Mr. SANFORD. Thank you, Mr. Chairman, and, again, thank you for holding this hearing. Thank the Ranking Member as well.

What I am hearing back home is that people are really concerned about the disconnect between what they see and what they hear. So, what they are hearing is it is not communicable. People are relatively safe. But meanwhile they are seeing pictures of people coming out of buildings wearing space suits, and what people are telling me back home is, I do not have a space suit, how am I safe? So there is a real disconnect between what they are seeing in terms of the imagery and what they are hearing.

I would also, though, follow up on the Chairman's point. It was your words, Mr. Merlin, just a few moments ago that this disease was "ferocious." Your words were that it was spreading exponentially, and it was the largest outbreak ever of Ebola. I asked our staff to look at, you know, how we treated some of these things in the past. One of the big benchmarks they used was the Spanish flu of 1918 which killed millions around the world, and the different protocols between New York City and at that time Pittsburgh, which were two of the bigger cities on the East Coast. New York immediately implemented quarantine. Pittsburgh waited a month, and as a result, very, very different results in terms of death in those respective cities, New York faring quite well relative to Pittsburgh.

So, what people have been saying to me back home is that, well, wait a minute, if this thing is as virulent as some folks suggest, why in the world of quarantine are we going to let people fly from that part of the world—and this is following up on the Chairman's question that he is getting from his constituents as well—to this part of the world? What you said just a moment ago was we need uninhibited travel, but last time I checked, the 101st Airborne, they do not fly on Delta. I mean, military air can get resources, people, health professionals in without having civilians going in and out.

Then the second thing you said was we want to prevent these countries from collapsing economically. I think that that overstates the case. I mean, from a U.S. standpoint, certainly what happens economically in Guinea or Sierra Leone is not going to drive the American economy and vice versa. From the opposite end, we have had a travel embargo with Cuba for about 50 years now. It has not crippled the country.

So, it seems to me, again, what a lot of people back home are saying to the Chairman's point and question is, why would you not just, you know, if you are over there, we are not going to issue a travel issue coming over here until we get this thing sorted out? Because going back to my colleague from Utah's question just a moment ago, it seems to me that there is a real mismatch between, well, CDC is saying, well, you know, Border Patrol folks have got it, and they are pointing to health care professionals. Until we get all that sorted out, why would you not just say let us just wait on travel right now?

Dr. MERLIN. Congressman, those are very good questions, and they are understandable questions. I have to admit that I wince every time I see the TV images with people in space suits because it gives an impression about the infectivity of the virus that is not realistic. It is an overreaction, and I think it flames people's fears about Ebola and how Ebola is spread. Doctors Without Borders has taken care of Ebola patients for years by using established personal protective equipment that does not include those sort of space suits that you see on television without acquiring infection in their workers. So, some of this is unfortunately media-driven.

As to the difference between the influenza epidemic of 1918 and Ebola, there are really major differences——

Mr. SANFORD. Understood, but I see we have gone to a yellow light, and we have a couple of seconds left. But why not, again, prohibition on civilian travel from this part of the world, that part of the world? If you are over there, do not come here. Why not?

Mr. WAGNER. We feel that that would cause the disease to grow in that area and to spill over into other countries, and then spill over more into the United States, and the real opportunity now is to put out that disease there. Every travel restriction that has been placed on travel into that area has interfered with people who are trying to help not being able to get there, either travel restrictions or reduction in air travel.

It is not just the U.S. military, you know. It is people from Europe. It is people from China. It is people from Cuba who are trying to get there to help. It would make doing what we need to do harder, and that is why we ask the American people's understanding of that.

Mr. SANFORD. I hear you. I have questions on that, but my time has expired. Thank you, Mr. Chairman.

Chairman MCCAUL. I thank the gentleman, and Mr. Barber is recognized.

Mr. BARBER. Thank you, Mr. Chairman, and thank you, Ranking Member Thompson, for convening this very important hearing today. People back home are concerned, and I came here to ask questions on their behalf as well as to get answers.

But before I do that, I just want to extend my condolences to Mr. Duncan's family and to all of the people in the countries that are affected. I think the video we have seen on television of the suffering in Africa just touches our hearts, and I know the United States is mobilizing to help. So, I commend our men and women in uniform for taking this mission on. I know they will do an incredible job building facilities to help care for those who are sick. I also, Commissioner Wagner, want to commend your men and women because you are really on the front line when it comes to how do we make sure that we control people coming in who might be bringing this disease to our country.

I appreciate what the Chairman said earlier about this not being a political issue, and we have to make sure we avoid making it one. This is an American issue for the safety of the people we represent, and it is an American issue for what we always do so well, and that is help other countries who are not able to do what they need to do for themselves.

I do hope, Mr. Chairman, as we look at what is needed here today that we as Members of Congress will return after the election fully committed to providing the funding that is necessary, to provide the resources that are necessary, for CDC and for our men and women who are trying to protect the Nation and address this disease.

I want to go to the question that has come up now a couple of times, Commissioner Wagner, about how it is that we control or manage travelers coming from the countries that are most affected today. I understand the concerns about stopping flights, but let me suggest another possible measure to you and get your reaction. Would it be helpful to require individuals who are not U.S. citizens or permanent residents traveling from the countries that are affected, to require them to go to the local American consulate or embassy in their respective countries to get a visa, and perhaps we could implement some screening at that location before people actually embark for the United States. Could you comment?

Mr. WAGNER. Well, they have to have a visa already to come here, part of that process. It does make a person inadmissible to the United States if you have any number of communicable diseases. Once they get that visa, if they develop that disease or that illness, upon entry into the United States, as part of our immigration authorities and admissibility questioning and inspection process, we will be alert for overt signs of illness of a person.

Mr. BARBER. Well, can I just interject, though? I appreciate that people have to have a visa. I guess what I was going at, and maybe this is a question for the State Department. Could we not implement at our consulates or embassies the same kind of screening procedures that you are implementing and perhaps even beyond what you are implementing at people coming into our country? It seems to me if we could catch the disease before it actually embarks, we would be in a much better place to protect the United States and the citizens of the United States.

Mr. WAGNER. Yes. I would have to defer to the Department of State on that one if everyone had to, say, reapply for a new visa subject to that level of condition.

Mr. BARBER. Well, let me turn next to Dr. Merlin. I just want to commend the CDC for taking on this incredible challenge. I have a lot of confidence in what the CDC does for our country. But I am also cognizant that unfortunately the CDC has been impacted heavily by budget cuts over the last several years, and I hope when we return, as I said earlier, we will take a look at what you need to make sure that this job is done with the resources that are needed.

You mentioned earlier, Dr. Merlin, that we have known about this disease for 30 years. I have one question as my time is running out. Is it not possible, and perhaps it is already underway, for us to develop a test that would understand the nature of the illness in an individual before we have to wait 21 days? Can we not examine that person in another way rather than waiting for the disease to be apparent?

Dr. MERLIN. Congressman Barber, that is an excellent question, and it comes up repeatedly. We have currently no diagnostic test that will detect Ebola before an individual develops symptoms. In fact, our current testing may not detect Ebola in the first 3 days of illness. If there is a patient who is suspected of having Ebola and the first test is negative, we often recommend a second test at 72 hours.

I think that is a good challenge, and it would be very helpful to have a test like that. Developing tests to perform on asymptomatic individuals is very difficult because you need to find a target. You need to find something that is distinctive and present enough in the infected individual and the non-infected individual. That is very hard to do.

Mr. BARBER. I appreciate it. Mr. Chairman, my time is up. Let me just close by saying I think we ought to redouble our efforts to do just such testing. I think it would be very useful to our efforts to control this disease. Thank you, Dr. Merlin.

Dr. MERLIN. I will take that back. Thank you.

Mr. BARBER. Thank you, Mr. Chairman.

Chairman MCCAUL. The Chairman now recognizes the gentleman from Florida, Mr. Clawson.

Mr. CLAWSON. Thank you for coming here today. Appreciate your service to our country, and I know how hard you all are working now to keep us safe. Thank you to the Ranking Member and Chairman for doing this committee meeting, particularly here in Dallas. Good job. We have great first responders in our country. Having lived large parts of my life overseas, I just think it is not comparable to anywhere else that I have seen. I want to congratulate you all on that, those of you involved in that, first of all, and really say it is a good job.

I am worried now about our first responders that are going to Africa, so my first question is to Dr. Merlin. You know, we are going to have 3,200 troops that are not medical experts in these mobile labs, as I understand it, doing testing and so forth. So my first question is to you all regarding that. Are our Good Samaritans going to be okay here? Are our Good Samaritans going to be safe? That is the first thing that popped in my mind. I have so many veterans in my district. Are our first responders going to be okay to go to Africa?

The second thing I wanted to ask is how long until we do have a vaccine? What will it take to get there? If I understood this morning you all saying this a highly infectious disease, Dr. Merlin, is that right? Fatal up to 90 percent? If I heard you right, not necessarily contagious like influenza. Okay. It sounds still pretty deadly. So, how far out is a vaccine?

Then my question to Mr. Wagner, you talked about the enhanced efforts, and you are going to get us more information on exactly procedurally what that means. How long until you are there? I remember after 9/11, it took us a while for TSA really to get up to speed, and they are a lot better at what they now than right after the disaster, and a similar analogy. How long until you think that you are confident that there are no holes in the security wall that is your force? If you all would answer these questions for me, I would really appreciate it.

Dr. MERLIN. Thank you, Congressman Clawson. The safety of anyone who we deploy in an epidemic like this is of utmost concern. We are putting people in harm's way by having them go to someplace where they might get infected. We, working with our partner organizations and DoD, do training and provide personal protective equipment or coordinate the use of personal protective equipment to keep people from getting infected. Our military forces are going to be not on a treatment mission. They are not going to be providing direct care, but they are going to be doing logistical work, but still it is a concern. We will do everything possible to prevent people who are trying to help from getting infected.

Mr. CLAWSON. I think the goal here is zero.

Dr. MERLIN. I agree. I agree completely. Now I am forgetting your second question.

Mr. CLAWSON. Vaccine.

Dr. MERLIN. Vaccine. You know, I would prefer that the National Institutes of Health, which is responsible for overseeing the vaccine development, and BARDA speak to the actual time tables for development. Fortunately, there are candidate vaccines available that have shown efficacy in non-human primates, but before administering those vaccines to people, you need to be absolutely sure that they do no harm to people when you administer them to people. Those trials are going on now. Then you have to know the right dose to administer, and you have to have the manufacturing capability.

I know that the agencies are working simultaneously to do those trials and ramp up the manufacturing capability. But both BARDA and NIH are better to testify on that than I am.

Mr. CLAWSON. Do those trials in these sorts of days of crisis, do those trials go to the top of the heap?

Dr. MERLIN. Yes.

Mr. CLAWSON. Because there is quite a backlog, as you know.

Dr. MERLIN. They have gone to the top of the heap. I can assure you of that.

Mr. CLAWSON. Thank you. Mr. Wagner.

Mr. WAGNER. Today we screen all travelers for any over signs of illness for a host of communicable diseases, from measles, to tuberculosis, to H1N1, to MERS, to SARS, you know, including, you know, symptoms of Ebola. What we are kicking off Saturday at JFK is some extended procedures about taking people's temperatures and asking them very specific questions about contact with people who have Ebola and then working closely with the CDC to get those people that answer affirmative or have a temperature in getting them into some professional medical care to address that.

All the other locations will continue to—I think we have four other locations—I am sorry—that will kick off following Saturday at some point next week. That will cover about 94 percent of all of the travelers to the United States coming from those three regions. All our other locations will continue to identify any travelers that go to those locations.

Mr. CLAWSON. Can I butt in real quick?

Mr. WAGNER. Yes.

Mr. CLAWSON. That means you are doing face-to-face training right now in those airports with those officers so that we will have an upgraded procedure starting almost immediately.

Mr. WAGNER. We have on-going training. We have an annual certification for all officers about blood-borne pathogens and diseases. Our Basic Training Academy covers a lot of the work with CDC and recognizing signs of illness and the protocols for handing that person off to CDC for the medical care. That is on-going and continuous. We have done that for a number of years going back to a lot of our pandemic planning with SARS, and MERS, and a lot of the other contagious illnesses out there.

Mr. CLAWSON. Thank you all three.

Chairman MCCAUL. The Chairman recognizes Mr. O'Rourke.

Mr. O'ROURKE. Thank you, Mr. Chairman. For Dr. Merlin, my understanding is that there are experimental treatments for Ebola, and that Mr. Duncan was diagnosed on the 30th of September, but did not receive treatment until the 4th of October. Give me your thoughts on that and whether or not that might have contributed to his death; in other words, the delay in his receiving that treatment.

Dr. MERLIN. Yes. The people who understand best the decision-making process around whether and when to administer experimental therapies to the patient are really the care team providing care for the patient, and the patient, and the patient's family. We at CDC, our job is to make the public health officials and the team aware of what experimental therapies are available and how to go about acquiring them. Sometimes we facilitate that, but we do not actually——

Mr. O'ROURKE. You do not have authority to order a specific treatment, so that would be a question better asked to the care team.

Dr. MERLIN. Exactly.

Mr. O'ROURKE. Let me then move on to my next question. We have talked a lot about airports and what we are doing to screen their capacity, training, protocols. What—from a public health perspective, and then I am going to ask Mr. Wagner from an operational perspective. What are the threats at our other ports of entry, sea ports and land ports, from a public health perspective?

Dr. MERLIN. We have had already a number of cargo ships that come in all the time with people who are sick on the ships. Often, you know, the Coast Guard is the sort-of first line of defense on that. They engage with the Coast Guard, and then usually with, I believe, with CBP and with us to determine what the best course of action is with the person on a ship.

This is more complicated because often there is a question of how long the person has been on the ship, and where the ship has been, and what the person's nature of exposure was. So these are harder cases to deal with, and they are also harder because often the person who is sick on the ship is gravely ill. It is a more difficult situation to deal with.

Mr. O'ROURKE. Mr. Wagner, what capacity do we have at these other ports to handle potentially infected travelers?

Mr. WAGNER. The land border is a lot more challenging because we do not have the advanced notice of the travelers' itinerary or their arrival. So, again, we would be alert for any overt signs of illness, and through our routine questioning——

Mr. O'ROURKE. CBP Officers at land ports are receiving that training to know now to look that?

Mr. WAGNER. Yes. Absolutely, yes, all our officers get that. So during their normal processing of a traveler, if they see these signs of illness, they have the contacts with CDC to get the medical professional advice on what to do and for follow-up for the traveler. But tuberculosis, measles, other communicable-type diseases, you know, we do see coming across the border.

Mr. O'ROURKE. My last question, again, for Dr. Merlin, CDC administers public health emergency preparedness grants, $640 million that go to all States. What concerns or questions do you have or answers for us about accountability for how that money is spent and used, especially given some of the mistakes made in Dallas with the handling of Mr. Duncan's case? What recommendations, if any, do you have going forward in terms of additional accountability and potentially additional resources if you feel that those are needed?

Dr. MERLIN. That is a very good question, Congressman. I think we need to assure that, and steps have already been taken in this, that the PHEP grant and the hospital preparedness grant programs are well-coordinated. That both grants assure that not only health departments, but facilities are well-prepared for potential and infectious disease emergencies, and that we sort-of have a seamless system.

You know, prior to about 2 years ago, the grants were administered independently, and now they are better-coordinated. But we need to be sure that the guidance is reaching the people in the facilities who will encounter the patient for the first time and they know how to respond, and that they are exercised. They are not simply protocols that are put away, that they are things that people know how to do.

Mr. O'ROURKE. We will submit for the record some questions that try to get to the root of this, whether that money is being well-spent right now or whether we have the appropriate accountability to ensure that we have the training in place, especially given some of the mistakes that were made. I would love to get your answers to those in a little more specificity. Thank you. With that, I yield back to the Chairman.

Chairman MCCAUL. The Chairman recognizes the former Chairman of the Energy and Commerce Committee, Mr. Barton.

Mr. BARTON. I am glad to be recognized, Mr. Chairman, and I am glad to be a junior member ad hoc of your committee today.

[Laughter.]

Chairman MCCAUL. We are glad to have you.

Mr. BARTON. You and Mr. Thompson are holding a good hearing, and I am glad to be a small part of it.

Mr. Chairman, I want to feed off of the very first question that you asked in your question period. I think this is a serious issue. It is obvious that people are affected by it. It is very obvious that people are concerned by it. Here in the North Texas region, it is real. We have had an Ebola case. An individual not from the area who was traveling to the area has contracted the disease and has died, so it is not academic.

But first and foremost, this should be treated, I think, as a public health issue. It is not an international diplomacy issue. It is not a foreign policy. It is not a civil rights issue. It is a public health issue. In the community that I actually live in, Ennis, Texas, about 3 years ago a teacher contracted tuberculosis, was teaching his class. One of his students contracted the disease.

When that became known, the Texas Department of Public Health, which is going to testify on the next panel, came into the school district, interviewed all of the students immediately in the class, quarantined some, monitored some, came down, held a public hearing that I helped facilitate. But that was treated immediately as a public health issue and dealt with in such a way that there were no other cases contracted of TB.

It really does not appear to me right now that we are treating this primarily as a public health issue. Dr. Merlin, in a direct response to Chairman McCaul about why we do not stop flights from these countries in Africa, your response was because we need to send people and supplies over there to combat the disease. Well, obviously that is something that needs to be done. But as Governor Sanford pointed out, you do not have to have commercial flights to send flights into a country.

If we were really treating this as a public health issue, why would we not immediately stop these flights, and then on a case-by-case basis send equipment and people as necessary, and on a case-by-case basis allow people to come out? Why do we have to have commercial flights that under the best of screening procedures that you have talked about, you are almost guaranteed mathematically to miss some people?

So with due respect, I do not accept that answer that we cannot stop flights simply because we need to get people in. Do you have a response to that—or maybe Dr. Brinsfield might want to respond, too.

Dr. MERLIN. Well, Mr. Barton, I understand, and our experience has been that when there are interruptions in air travel, it impedes the public health response. Although there might be work-arounds, like military transport, that is difficult, and right now, time is of the essence in what we do.

Mr. BARTON. Well, who makes that decision? Is that a Presidential decision? Is that a Secretary of State decision? Is that a Secretary of Homeland Security decision? Who makes that decision about banning flights?

Dr. BRINSFIELD. So, sir, I would just like to point out, and I will defer to Chief Wagner here, that there are no direct flights from those areas, so that it is more an issue of what people are on flights coming from the intermediate airports.

Mr. WAGNER. Correct. So there are no direct flights from those three affected regions. These travelers are going to Brussels, Ghana, London, Paris, and Morocco to come here, and it may just be a couple of people on a single flight of 300 or 350 people. You may have——

Mr. BARTON. Well, you could still ban it. I mean, you could still. The gentleman who came from Liberia through, I believe, Brussels, he could have been stopped in Brussels or not even allowed a visa to leave to go to Brussels.

Dr. BRINSFIELD. I think that is the most important point, sir. At that point we defer to our colleagues at State, and there is a good coordination process around those questions.

Mr. BARTON. But my question on the table is: Who makes the decision? Is it the President, or the Secretary of State, or the Homeland Security, or who makes that decision?

Dr. BRINSFIELD. Sir, I would defer to the interagency process that is on-going under the President on this one.

Mr. BARTON. So it is the President?

Dr. BRINSFIELD. I would say that there are many different actions that you have discussed here, one related to visas, one related to flights landing. Those are different authorities. If the Department of State or Department——

Mr. BARTON. I know my time is expired, Mr. Chairman. Could a Governor of a State or could an airport authority ban flights from a particular region, or that has to be done at the Federal level?

Mr. WAGNER. Sir, most of the airports are landing rights airports, and they request permission from Customs and Border Protection to land. So I think it is a question more for the airlines and the airport authorities on what business they choose to do or not do.

Mr. BARTON. So theoretically DFW Airport could ban a flight from a passenger coming——

Mr. WAGNER. I would have to defer to them on what business decisions they make and where to fly to and which airlines they go to.

Mr. BARTON. Thank you, Mr. Chairman, for your courtesy.

Chairman MCCAUL. Thank you. The Chairman recognizes Mr. Vela from Texas.

Mr. VELA. Thank you, Mr. Chairman. Dr. Merlin, I am trying to understand, what is the scientific explanation for the response that a travel ban would actually make things worse?

Dr. MERLIN. Mr. Vela, thank you for asking that question. We have a disease now that we understand the range of how many people are infected. We know how many people would be infected next month if nothing is done, and how many people will be infected by the end of the year if nothing is done. We know the size and the scale of the international effort. It is a remarkable international effort that is required to stop it.

We have good projections on how many deaths will be caused by delay, and we are very afraid that things that are done that impede travel will delay the interventions that prevent the progression of the disease. If the disease progresses to the point that it cannot be stopped, it is going to spill over into other countries and create a greater threat for the United States.

So we feel that understandably the notion of stopping travelers now might prevent a traveler from arriving in the United States, though we know we can prevent an outbreak from that. But the greater risk is that by delaying stopping the epidemic in Guinea, Sierra Leone, and Liberia, you create a much larger epidemic that is impossible to control. That disease becomes endemic in Africa, and that we are dealing with this for the foreseeable future, that we cannot stop it. What we want to do is stop it right now. We know how to do it. We just need to get the resources there to do it. We do not want to do things that would impede that.

Mr. VELA. It also seems to me that there are two great risks, and that is the spread of the disease outside those three countries, and then following up a point Mr. Wagner was making from the flight standpoint, from people who are traveling from those three countries anywhere else.

What kind of international coordination are we seeing, and I was wondering if you could maybe give us an idea. I mean, who is helping us? What is the international community doing to stop the spread of the virus into the other adjacent countries, and from going to airports, like Brussels and any other point in between?

Dr. MERLIN. I can tell you from a public health perspective, CDC regards this as a very high priority. We have over 140 individuals deployed to not only Sierra Leone, Guinea, and Liberia, but neighboring countries where they are involved in working with the ministries of health and training individuals so that they know how to detect disease early and engage in contact tracing and break the transmission of disease.

So what we want to happen in those countries is when an ember of the disease lands in their country and starts a fire, for them to be able to quench the disease as quickly as possible, and that is the sort of public health approach. I do not know about the air travel issue, and I would defer to my colleagues. They may know about the coordination of air travel.

Dr. BRINSFIELD. I would just say that the response is well-coordinated under the United Nations and has been for several weeks. I would defer questions on follow-up on the international response to them and their Department of State partners.

Mr. VELA. Let me ask you this question. Aside from the hemorrhaging, the symptoms of the virus appear very similar to any severe flu. Are there any other distinctions?

Dr. MERLIN. In clinical presentation, early clinical presentation, no. It is unfortunate that it has the name of viral hemorrhagic fever because only a minority of patients develop bleeding symptoms, and that is late in the course of the disease. So early in the course of the disease, the first 3 days, it is a flu-like illness. It is fever, malaise. There is nothing about the clinical presentation that would make you know it was Ebola. After about 3 days, there is usually profound nausea, vomiting, and diarrhea, and that is what my colleagues and I, when we hear stories about people presenting, that what really raises the flag that this might be Ebola.

So the travel history and exposure history are very important to include with the early symptoms to understand where someone might actually have Ebola. You cannot tell just on the symptoms alone. You need more information.

Mr. VELA. Is my time up? Thank you.

Chairman MCCAUL. The Chairman recognizes Dr. Burgess, who actually practiced at Dallas Presbyterian Hospital.

Mr. BURGESS. Thank you, Mr. Chairman, and I thank our panel for being here. Dr. Brinsfield, Mr. Wagner, appreciate you all spending time with me on the telephone earlier this week. It was very helpful, and I am sure we will continue to have discussions as this story evolves.

We are appropriately respectful of the passing of Mr. Duncan. I think we also ought to acknowledge the passing of Patrick Sawyer at the end of July. Mr. Sawyer was an individual who worked in Liberia, commuted to there from his home in Minneapolis. After attending his ill sister in Liberia, flew on to Lagos. Before he could board the plane back to Minneapolis died of Ebola, and could have been Patient Zero 2 months before we had the experience here.

So, Dr. Merlin, I guess my question is, I am sure there will be after-action reports on the case that occurred here in Dallas. Did you do any study of what might have happened had Patient Zero arrived in Minneapolis on July 30?

Dr. MERLIN. Congressman Burgess, I am not aware of that, and I will have to get back to you on that. I do not know.

Mr. BURGESS. Well, the reason I asked the question, and Ms. Jackson Lee, I think, put it pretty clearly, you have a situation at Presbyterian. A nurse does an intake evaluation, and apparently some travel history is given that perhaps provided a really important clue that was subsequently lost in all of the activities involved with treating the individual. From the CDC standpoint, are you concerned at all with the directives and missives and action alerts that you have putting out for months that somehow they were not getting through to the front line, to the people at the triage desk? Because really there was only one response: I am here for a fever and a stomach ache. I have traveled from Africa. Put down the iPad. Go through that door with the two men in moon suits. We will meet you and walk you into an isolation unit. Really that is the only response; is that not correct?

Dr. MERLIN. Congressman Burgess, I agree with you. As someone who has worked in a hospital and in an emergency room, I am sure you know that things in retrospect are often a lot clearer than they are when present.

Mr. BURGESS. But from a CDC perspective, you have put out these directives to the hospitals, to the people on the front lines. You know, this is not the flu as usual. You have got to be thinking about this. If I am at CDC, I have to be concerned that that message did not get down to the front line. Not to be critical of anyone. Not to be accusatory of anyone. But the message did not get to the front line. What are you going to do now differently to make sure that message does get to the people on the front line, because that is really the critical part that was missed?

Dr. MERLIN. I think what we need to do is to work with the regulatory organizations, like the Joint Commission, to be sure that compliance with preparedness is a higher priority, and that when facilities are accredited, that it is something that is looked at critically, and they look at whether the front line is trained on these things.

Mr. BURGESS. I would just offer that business as usual may not get it because this is not an ordinary time with what we are dealing with.

Now, two airlines, Air France and British Airways, stopped going to Monrovia in the summer, I think in August. So they just simply on their own decided they were going to stop service there. I know people have asked me. The President actually suspended air operations through the FAA into the airport in Israel for a while this summer while there was some bombing going on, so we know that authority exists.

Okay. Mr. Thompson provided this nice graph, and Dr. Brinsfield, you will recognize this graph. This is a classic growth curve. You have got a lag phase. You have got a log phase, the log phase, the phase of logarithmic growth, the exponential phase. In two countries at least it appears—Sierra Leone and Liberia—they are in the logarithmic phase. Dr. Fouts, he said in another hearing that I was at in Washington a few weeks ago that when you get to logarithmic, when you get to exponential growth, exponential always wins.

So my question is: Where on this line is the threat matrix such that you would recommend to the President we have got to do something different, and we have got to stop this disease, and not allow it to be imported to our country, but this does not come in through a migratory flyway? It is not like pandemic flu. You can only get Ebola if you go get it and then bring it home. So where is the point on this graph where that would occur?

Dr. MERLIN. We are already at the point where we believe that all stops needs to be pulled out in preventing the growth of the disease in Africa, and that is what we need to focus on because the risk in this country will not be eliminated until we eliminate the spread of disease in Africa.

I think that comes down to the crucial point is that we will not be safe until we stop the growth of that disease because it has now infected so many people, and it is reproducing so quickly that unless we stop it, it will inevitably become endemic, and it will inevitably be a greater threat. So I think the President has already taken the message out to the American people and to the United Nations that this is the time. The opportunity space is right now.

Mr. BURGESS. Dr. Merlin, I know my time is up. With all due respect, I disagree with you. I do not think the President has put a significant amount of importance on this. I have not heard the President say this is the time of zero defects. We have got to do everything perfectly. Doctors Without Borders, that has been their experience over in those countries. They have a low infection rate even though health care workers have a high infection rate because they do everything by the book every time, and we need to adopt that same attitude here.

Thank you, Mr. Chairman. You are very kind.

Chairman MCCAUL. The gentleman's time has expired. The Chairman recognizes Mr. Swalwell form California.

Mr. SWALWELL. Thank you, Mr. Chairman, and thank you to our panelists. What I have taken away from this hearing and what we have learned over the past month is we have to fight this aggressively, and, most importantly, over in the countries involved in West Africa. To that, we have to be prepared here locally, whether it is the airport screens that take place or the hospitals that are ready. Also, No. 3, that we have to bust some of the myths out there that are creating, I think, unnecessary hysteria.

So I want to first start with what we can do here locally with the airport screens. Mr. Wagner, we know that every day about 1.75 million people are in the air in the United States. We have about 100,000 pilots, 95,000 flight attendants who are on the front lines who could be exposed to this. I think some good questions are rightfully being asked.

So, one of my concerns, although we have five airports that are now going to have intensified screenings, what would happen if somebody were to fly from, say, Brussels to Dallas-Fort Worth Airport, and then, like many foreign travelers, stuck around in the United States for 2 to 3 weeks and went from Dallas-Fort Worth to, say, San Francisco International Airport? That is not one of the five designated airports. Would that person who perhaps did not present symptoms at DFW, but started to present symptoms as they went into San Francisco, is there anything there that would allow us to screen that individual?

Mr. WAGNER. Well, Customs and Border Protection is only going to screen them on their initial entry into the United States. So when we see them coming into DFW, we would identify that travel as having originated in one of those three areas. We would have provided them the information notice about symptoms to watch out for and where to go and seek help. The information notice also has a message to the doctor that they can provide. But then we are relying on that person wherever they travel within the United States, if they start to develop those symptoms, they need to go get the proper medical care and get the medical authorities to make that determination that is it Ebola or is the flu or is it something else.

Mr. SWALWELL. Sure. Dr. Merlin, as far as our local hospitals, I am having a conference call with all of our hospital officials on Tuesday. What are we doing to reach out to them to make sure that they know what to look for if a patient comes in and has been traveling to some of these West Africa countries and is presenting symptoms?

Dr. MERLIN. We have been communicating with hospitals through a variety of mechanisms. We have an established email electronic communication, a health alert network, that goes to thousands of facilities and providers in the country. We have been working with our State and local partners to reach out to facilities and physicians. We have a regular conference call called the COCA call, which is a clinical outreach call, where I believe one of the ones recently on Ebola had about 6,000 participants on it.

We have been working through the medical societies. There were a lot of presentations. This is Infectious Disease Week, and the Infectious Disease Society of America just had its meetings, and there were a lot of presentations on Ebola. We have a large group in our Emergency Operations Center that regularly now is having outreach calls to either individual hospitals that want questions answered or professional groups that want to have questions answered. We have had conference calls from, you know, single facilities to large groups of facilities trying to help them with their preparations.

Mr. SWALWELL. Dr. Merlin, my colleague, Mr. Barber from Arizona, alluded to the CDC budget, and budgets reflect priorities and values. I think the numbers around the CDC budget over the past few years reflect that prioritizing public health and addressing world-wide health emergencies have not been our top priority when it comes to the numbers.

From 2010 to 2014, the CDC budget has steadily gone down. From 2012 to 2013, the program level for the CDC was cut by $293 million, which included $13 million in cuts to our efforts to prevent and respond to outbreaks of emerging infectious diseases. Is today's funding level for the CDC adequate to address the world-wide threat and what could happen here in the United States? Would you like more, and if you had more, what would you do with it?

Dr. MERLIN. The response to that I would defer to the CDC director and HHS. I am not in the position at CDC where I really understand and participate in the full budget formulation.

Mr. SWALWELL. Has your budget been cut, though, since sequestration?

Dr. MERLIN. I will have to get back to you on that. My budget comes from multiple different sources, and I would have to get back to you on that.

Mr. SWALWELL. Sure. Thank you, Mr. Chairman, and I yield back.

Chairman MCCAUL. The Chairman now recognizes the gentleman from Texas, Mr. Marchant.

Mr. MARCHANT. I would like to thank the Chairman today for holding this hearing and welcome all the Congressmen to my district. This is the heart of my Congressional district. It is the economic hub. Thousands of my constituents come to work every day in this district, and as you know, 5 million international travelers come through this airport every year.

So in response to that, I would like to submit for the record a letter to the Honorable Jeh Johnson that I made this morning asking for Dallas-Fort Worth International Airport to be included or added to the list of five airports that are going to have the increased screening and a letter from the Dallas-Fort Worth International Airport.

Chairman MCCAUL. Without objection, so ordered.

[The information follows:]

LETTER SUBMITTED FOR THE RECORD BY HONORABLE KENNY MARCHANT

OCTOBER 9, 2014.

The Honorable JEH JOHNSON,
Secretary, Department of Homeland Security, Washington, DC 20528.

DEAR SECRETARY JOHNSON: I am writing to strongly call for the immediate inclusion of Dallas/Fort Worth (DFW) International Airport—which I represent in Congress—in the list of other major U.S. airports at which the administration has announced it will implement heightened Ebola-related security screening protocols. DFW Airport is the third busiest airport in the world, hosting over 1,800 flights per day and serving more than 62 million passengers each year. As you are aware, it was also the final U.S. arrival destination of Thomas Eric Duncan, the first individual diagnosed with Ebola inside the United States. Action must be taken to ensure that the people of North Texas do not suffer greater exposure to this deadly virus.

The White House has said that five U.S. airports receive roughly 94% of the roughly 150 passengers from the three affected countries that arrive in the U.S. each day. What risk do the remaining 6% of passengers have on major airports, such as DFW, that have not been selected for additional screening? How difficult would be it for Customs to review the additional 6% of passengers, which amounts to approximately 9 people per day? The administration should execute every defense against persons and materials entering the U.S. to guard against any new Ebola cases arriving in the United States.

Thank you for your review of this correspondence. Should you have any questions regarding this letter, please feel free to contact me or my Legislative Director.

Sincerely,

KENNY MARCHANT,
Member of Congress.

————

LETTER FROM THE DALLAS/FORT WORTH INTERNATIONAL AIRPORT SUBMITTED FOR THE RECORD BY HONORABLE KENNY MARCHANT

OCTOBER 7, 2014.

The Honorable KENNY MARCHANT,
Member of Congress, 24th District, Texas, 1110 Longworth House Office Building, Washington, DC 20515.

DEAR CONGRESSMAN MARCHANT: Dallas/Fort Worth International Airport (DFW) appreciates your concern and your leadership on behalf of our country and your constituents. In response to your recent letter, I want to assure you that the Airport takes our responsibility for the safety and security of customers, passengers and employees very seriously. DFW's role in response to infectious disease is that of first responder to any report of anyone at the Airport who exhibits signs or symptoms consistent with any communicable disease. DFW has in place a robust and exercised pandemic response plan that has been reviewed by all relevant agencies.

With regard to infectious disease control and our country's pandemic response, DFW is part of an integrated response system under the direction of the Centers for Disease Control and Prevention (CDC) and local public health authorities.

We rigorously adhere to the guidelines of the CDC which has jurisdiction in the matter of infectious disease control. As such, procedures and protocols are in place to ensure that DFW effectively responds to reports of infectious disease by U.S. Customs and Border Protection (CBP) as individuals are entering the country, by airlines for passengers or employees who show symptoms of infectious diseases of many types, as well as reports from other segments of the travel industry and public health community.

In addition to the CDC, in the case of our terminals, we follow the direction of the Tarrant County Department of Public Health, which is also responsible for public communication.

DFW will continue to take direction and guidance from the CDC and our federal government with regard to any additional safety and security measures deemed necessary to protect the safety and security of our country and the traveling public.
Sincerely,

SEAN DONOHUE,
Chief Executive Officer, DFW International Airport.

Mr. MARCHANT. Thank you. Mr. Wagner, there are approximately 13,500 people from the affected areas that have travel visas that are active at this point. What Federal agency is responsible for knowing who those 13,500 people are and the status of their travel?

Mr. WAGNER. Well, the Department of State issues that visa, so they would be responsible for who has them and under what conditions. Customs and Border Protection would encounter that individual when they arrive to the United States. Part of what we determine in that inspection process is does that person intend to comply with the terms of that visa, and then are there any grounds for inadmissibility, such as a communicable illness, that would prevent them from coming in?

Mr. MARCHANT. So if we indeed are at a critical point in containing this disease, do you not think it is important or would you not think that it is important that there be some identifiable base of people that have come through Customs and Border Protection that are in the United States or have traveled in the United States that have presented their passport, have been questioned, have been screened, and so that we have some idea of what the number is? I mean, how many people could this possibly have affected?

Mr. WAGNER. Well, we would know how many people came into the United States from those affected regions over the course of, you know, any period of time. You know, where they are in the United States, or who they have had contact with, or what has, you know, transpired since then is a much more complex issue.

Mr. MARCHANT. So DFW Airport is not usually the primary point of entry for these countries, but as most people across the country know, if you go anywhere in the United States, you are probably going to have to go through DFW Airport. I think it is very critical at this point that we understand that people are coming into JFK and they are coming into Newark and these other five entry points and staying 1 or 2 or 3 weeks or 4 weeks, and then they are coming through DFW Airport, and they are going all over the country.

So I think this is a key place where we need to have an active program of screening going on. Do we have a CDC facility that is close? Are we are one of the 20 areas where the CDC has a center?

Dr. MERLIN. No, we do not have a staffed facility at DFW. We may have a physical space, but it is not currently staffed.

Mr. MARCHANT. Mr. Chairman, I would like to request that the CDC strongly consider DFW Airport, as well as George Bush International in Texas, and fully staffing those. Our Governor has just recently asked questions about whether our CDC facilities—where they were located and how well they are staffed.

Chairman MCCAUL. Without objection. Just for the record, I submitted a letter along with Senator Cornyn to the Secretary asking the same request. I'll include it also. So ordered.

[The information follows:]

LETTER FROM CHAIRMAN MICHAEL T. MCCAUL AND SENATOR JOHN CORNYN

OCTOBER 10, 2014.

R. GILL KERLIKOWSKE,
Commissioner, U.S. Customs and Border Protection, Washington, D.C.

DEAR COMMISSIONER KERLIKOWSKE: We are writing about the decision by the Department of Homeland Security to provide enhanced screening to passengers from the Ebola-affected nations of Guinea, Liberia, and Sierra Leone.

As you may know, Texas is home to both Houston George Bush Intercontinental Airport (IAH) and Dallas-Fort Worth International Airport (DFW) where a combined 15.6 million international passengers visited in 2013. Neither airport has been designated for enhanced screening. Because those traveling from Guinea, Sierra Leone, and Liberia can transit to the United States from many other countries, we have concerns that the current decision to screen only at five airports may not adequately protect Americans and others traveling to America from the Ebola virus.

Therefore, we request that you provide answers to the following questions:

(1) According the Administration, the enhanced screening will take place at five airports that receive 94 percent of the passengers from the three affected countries. Where do the other 6 percent arrive? Will other major international airports be designated for enhanced screening procedures and additional resources if this limited initiative does not effectively mitigate against entry of potentially infected passengers?

(2) How many from those Ebola-affected countries enter the United States through other ports of entry, such as sea ports and land border stations?

(3) What other Ebola-related measures are being taken at other vulnerable port environments, particularly at high traffic land border ports of entry along the Texas-Mexico border? If none, why? Will U.S. Border Patrol apply enhanced screening procedures to those apprehended between land border ports of entry?

(4) Please explain the tracking system in place for those traveling from Liberia, Guinea, and Sierra Leone to the U.S. How are you working with other countries that have connecting flights from West Africa to the U.S. to ensure an adequate screening process?

(5) What passenger travel documentation do Customs and Border Protection Officers inspect when a passenger arrives in the U.S.? Is documentation other than the origin and connection of the passenger available for inspection?

We ask that you consider adding IAH and DFW to the list of airports performing enhanced screening.

Thank you for your attention to this matter. We look forward to a prompt reply.

Sincerely,

JOHN CORNYN,
UNITED STATES SENATOR.
MICHAEL T. MCCAUL,
United States Representative.

Mr. MARCHANT. Thank you, sir.

Ms. JACKSON LEE. Mr. Chairman, does that include Bush Intercontinental?

Chairman MCCAUL. I would have to look at the letter again, but I would concur with that as well.

Ms. JACKSON LEE. Thank you, Mr. Chairman.

Mr. MARCHANT. Mr. Chairman, I yield back my time.

Chairman MCCAUL. The Chairman now recognizes Mr. Veasey from Texas. I am sorry, Ms. Johnson, Eddie Bernice Johnson.

Ms. JOHNSON. Thank you very much, Mr. Chairman. My usual appreciation for all of the people that are here, and all of the respondees to this particular crisis.

Being a nurse, my concern really will center on the details of why we are in this position. It would seem to me, and I know that CDC had put protocols in every major hospital in this country for a number of weeks prior to this happening. So, no matter what else we do, we have got to depend on people that we question and whether or not they give the correct information.

I know we are talking about taking temperatures, and I do not know what other type of interrogation that they will have. But it would seem to me that we could not sit here and plan for the expenditure of a whole lot money that we are not going to do when we get back to Washington, but look very closely at what we have in place already, and to make sure that is given the kind of attention it demands to make it work.

Now, I do not know what questions were asked when this man went to the hospital the first time, nor do I know what temperature he had. But it would seem to me that much of what we are worried about right now could have been eliminated because the protocols were in place. Now, I do not know what happened with the protocols. But no matter how much we do to look at every person coming in this country, we have also got to carry out our own written protocols when they get here.

So, I am concerned about us sitting here and thinking about all the elaborate things we can do to make things better when we know we are not going to pay for it when we go back to Washington. We have not yet. We do not have the money. We do not have any more now than we did before we did it. So, I am concerned that we not get too much pie-in-the-sky in planning, but rather utilize what we have in place. Was there any faltering in the protocols that were in place?

Dr. MERLIN. Ms. Johnson, in terms of the adherence to protocols and what would have happened at Presbyterian Hospital, I really defer to the hospital itself and the local health department, the local and State Health Department. They are the ones who are responsible for reviewing that. I would not want to say things because I do not know the details.

Ms. JOHNSON. Yes.

Dr. MERLIN. But I do want to say to your point I think it is important to move from things like protocols to things like checklists where every patient in order to process through the facility, there has to be a checklist and they have to check off and sign whether they have done this, because that takes the protocol and makes it a firm responsibility. For things important like this, we really need to do it. That is one approach that I do not think adds much in the way of burden and assures better compliance with recommendations.

Ms. JOHNSON. Thank you very much. Mr. Wagner, what are we going to be doing differently than what we did when the patient entered this country? Was he not asked questions?

Mr. WAGNER. So if he were to enter through Dulles next week at some point, we will set up some enhanced level of screening. So we will have identified him as traveling from one of the affected regions. We would have given him a questionnaire to fill out that we work with CDC that talks about their contact information, their health status, do they have any symptoms in place, and, most importantly probably in this case, have they had any contact with anyone that has had Ebola. We would then also refer them to a medical professional on site to have their temperature taken.

If there any indications through that information that they need additional medical professional review, we would then coordinate with CDC on site to be able to have that.

Ms. JOHNSON. Can it not be assumed that someone comes in from Liberia that they have been in contact?

Dr. MERLIN. No. Our questions about contact really have to do not with being around or in an area that is infected, but really particularly whether someone has had contact exposure to body fluids. Have they had a splash of body fluids, with their unprotected hands touched body fluids? Have they have known a person who was known to have Ebola? Have they been for an extended period of time around someone who was known to have Ebola?

One of the things that we know about the disease in places like Liberia is it is actually patchy. There are places where there is a lot of disease, and there are places where there is very little disease. Our strategy out there, you know, is to actually prevent it from beginning to spread all over the place. We would not say in our public health line people from those countries have had contact with the disease.

Ms. JOHNSON. Well then, how would you determine an origin? If you cannot assume or at least act as if it is a possibility coming from those areas where it is very prominent, how would you draw the line from wherever they are coming from?

Dr. MERLIN. You know, your question is excellent and I think it ties into the question earlier about the test for a symptomatic disease. There is no objective test. We rely on examination, a visual, looking at the person, trying to tell whether the person might be ill, and a person's answering a series of questions to see whether the answers to the questions make sense. But that is the nature of the examination. Mr. Wagner, do you——

Ms. JOHNSON. Thank you—excuse me. Did I miss something?

Chairman MCCAUL. If we can make it brief, yes.

Mr. WAGNER. No, that is correct. It depends on how the people answer the questions and what they say to any follow-up questions we would ask.

Ms. JOHNSON. Thank you, Mr. Chairman. My time has expired.

Chairman MCCAUL. Of course, Mr. Duncan did not reveal that he had been in contact with the Ebola virus in Liberia, is that correct?

Mr. WAGNER. I believe so. I am not sure if he was aware——

Chairman MCCAUL. Dr. Merlin.

Dr. MERLIN. He did not truthfully answer the questions on the exit screening where he was asked whether he had an exposure. It turned out subsequently that he had a known exposure.

Chairman MCCAUL. The Chairman now recognizes Mr. Farenthold.

Mr. FARENTHOLD. Thank you very much. I am going to clean up here. I am going to have a bunch of quick questions, and if you could keep your answers relatively short. A lot of this is follow-ups on other questions.

I do want to say we have got to be real careful here. I do not think we are doing enough. If this disease gets a foothold in the United States, we take away the diagnostic question of have you been in these affected countries, so I think it is absolutely critical. I do not think we are doing enough.

Let me start with you, Mr. Wagner. We picked five airports to do. We learned that Mr. Duncan was less than truthful on his screening. We have just announced to the world what airports not to go through if you want to come to the United States because we have got better treatment. Could we maybe do something like funneling everybody who has a visa from one of these countries or who has traveled from one of these countries through one of the airports? Is that a step at least in the right direction? I think maybe banning all the flights is a right step, but is an intermediate step funneling everybody through the airport and screening?

Mr. WAGNER. I do not know that we can do that. I think it, again, relies on who the airlines choose to bring to us from different parts of the world.

Mr. FARENTHOLD. So we do not have the authority to say if you are coming from this country you can only enter through this port?

Mr. WAGNER. I do not believe so. I will have to look at that.

Mr. FARENTHOLD. If not, that is something we might be able to fix. Let me ask you another question, Mr. Wagner. You talked about how you all have the authority to stop people for health reasons. How often does that happen? Do you stop one person a day? I mean, it seems to me I do not ever hear about it on the news. Is it a frequent occurrence that you stop people?

Mr. WAGNER. We have a million people coming into the United States every day, so I would say it is not frequent, but it happens several times a week. You know, we have——

Mr. FARENTHOLD. All right. So you have less than a 1 in a million chance of getting——

Mr. WAGNER. No, I think it is who we have been advised that have a communicable disease, and we do get information about that and put it in our computer systems and are able to recognize that, I mean, and stop them from coming in.

Mr. FARENTHOLD. Right. But even now somebody that is not showing any symptoms is going to get through.

Mr. WAGNER. Well, if they are not showing any overt symptoms, it is tough for us to be able to recognize that they would be sick or have a disease that is, you know, to emerge in them. So I am not sure how——

Mr. FARENTHOLD. I understand. Listen, I do not want to shed all my rights to international travel any more than anyone else does, but we have got the obvious countries that we really need to be suspect of. Short of an absolute travel ban on these countries or canceling commercial flights, you know, an interim step is substantially enhanced screening and maybe follow-up screening every few days after they arrive.

I see, Mr. Merlin, you are nodding your head, but I have a couple of questions for you. I am sorry if I am skeptical of you and some of the things that you are saying. The American people and my constituents have lost trust in the Government for a variety of reasons, and I do not want to bring politics into public health. But we have the lowest level of trust in the Government, I think, in my memory. Add to that, every outbreak novel or zombie movie you see starts with somebody from the Government sitting in front of a panel like this saying there is nothing to worry about.

So you have got to remember the first two Ebola patients that came back to the United States were American doctors who became infected, who had all the training in the world and were Ebola experts. So my constituents, and to some degree I am, a little skeptical of the statement, oh, actually if you take the precautions it is very difficult to get. How did these two doctors get it, American-trained doctors? How did they come up with it in the first place if it is that difficult to get it, if our health care workers and the American public is safe?

Dr. MERLIN. Let me clarify for you what I said. For people who are health care workers who are putting themselves in environments where there are patients known to be infected with Ebola who have copious body fluids in the environment that carry the virus, the people have to practice scrupulously-known procedures for preventing acquisition of the virus. It is a dangerous environment in which to work, and it can only be done by scrupulous adherence to those precautions and caretaking measures.

Outside of those environments, when you are talking about a situation like the United States where we have a very sophisticated health care system and a sophisticated public health system, when we identify a case, we are capable of doing, what we have done with Mr. Duncan and we do with any future case, is assuring in collaboration with local and State health officials and the hospital community that the case is isolated and treated, that all contacts are quickly identified, and aggressively identified. If contacts are not reliable, that steps are taken to be sure that the contacts can be followed, that their temperatures are monitored. If they should become symptomatic, they are immediately hospitalized.

We know this works. It works in the United States, and it worked in Nigeria, and it worked in Senegal, so we can stop cases like that. Hopefully the difference between the zombie films and this testimony is this is real.

Mr. FARENTHOLD. I hope so. I see my time has expired, and I wish you the best of success in your efforts to contain this both in Africa and here in America.

Chairman MCCAUL. The Chairman now recognizes Mr. Veasey.

Mr. VEASEY. Thank you, Mr. Chairman. I want to ask Dr. Merlin a question. A second ago you said that it appeared that Mr. Duncan may have, you know, deceived the screeners at the airport. But I am looking at this memo that was prepared for the committee, and let me read you this and maybe see, is there something that needs to be clarified. "Although it is now believed that Mr. Duncan contracted the virus while helping a pregnant woman to the hospital, reports indicate that the woman's family told neighbors she was suffering from malaria, a disease with similar symptoms, not Ebola. Accordingly, there is no proof that Mr. Duncan intended to deceive airport screener on his questionnaire."

Dr. MERLIN. That is a fair question, and maybe we need to relook at the questionnaire to see what the language is. I am skeptical myself, and there is no way to know. There is no way to ask Mr. Duncan. I am skeptical that with Ebola well-established in Monrovia. I believe this woman he assisted was being taken to an Ebola hospital for treatment of Ebola, and she was turned away, and this is my understanding, and we can probably try to find out the facts on this. I am skeptical that he actually thought she had malaria.

But, you know, to your point, if we are asking whether you have been exposed to Ebola, it may have to be have you been exposed to anyone who has died of an infectious disease in the last period of time, because we need to be sure that we are not overly permissive in the questions.

Mr. VEASEY. Also let me get your opinion, again, on how the disease is spread. Is it your opinion that it would be highly unlikely that the disease would be spread through spit or sputum, or if someone sneezed or coughed, or, you know, for instance, in airline travel, bodily fluids inside of a lavatory?

Dr. MERLIN. In advanced Ebola disease, all bodily fluids are highly infectious. For someone with advanced disease, I think all of those materials would be highly infectious.

Mr. VEASEY. Including coughing and sneezing?

Dr. MERLIN. Well, you know, coughing, I mean, you would basically have to get the splatter into your face or into your eyes for it to be infectious. But I want to emphasize that people who are traveling, on exit screening, they have had their temperatures taken, so they are asymptomatic when they board the airlines. They are not going to do develop advanced disease on the 8- to 12-hour or 18-hour flight, so there is no risk that there is going to be an exposure on aircraft to someone with highly-infectious bodily fluids like that. That is just not going to happen.

Mr. VEASEY. But if someone could transmit Ebola through a conversation, and you do not have on a hazmat suit, if there is spit or sputum that is put in someone's eye through a conversation, which happens in normal conversations. So are you telling us that that would be a way to——

Dr. MERLIN. Yes, but, you know, people who are in close contact with someone with advanced disease are at risk. I want to emphasize that people who have no symptoms pose no risk to anyone. So the asymptomatic individual who coughs and speaks poses no risk. Someone who develops symptoms early in disease, which is the fever and fluid, they are not highly infectious. It is only late in disease. Now, if you are caring for someone who has advanced disease, and they cough on you, and they get the fluid in your face, yes, that is a risk.

Mr. VEASEY. Okay. One more question before my time expires here. Should we be concerned about other strands of the Ebola virus? I know you talked earlier about different strands. Should we be concerned about other strands of Ebola?

Dr. MERLIN. There are several species of Ebola virus. We are now dealing with Ebola Zaire. Yes, we do need to be concerned in Africa about all of the other species where they are and other outbreaks of Ebola Zaire to be sure that they are contained because most of them can cause very severe disease. So, yes, we do need to be concerned about the other strains.

Mr. VEASEY. Thank you, Mr. Chairman.

Chairman MCCAUL. I thank the witnesses for their testimony. This has been very valuable to the American people, and we support you and wish you all the best in your efforts to control and contain this horrific virus.

This panel is now dismissed. The clerk will prepare the witness table for our second panel.

[Recess.]

Chairman MCCAUL. We are ready to begin our second panel. First, we have Dr. David Lakey. He served as the commissioner of the Texas Department of State Health Services, leading one of the State's largest agencies with a staff of 11,500. He oversees programs such as disease prevention and bioterrorism preparedness, family and community health services, and many others.

Next, we have Dr. Brett Giroir. He assumed leadership of the Texas A&M Science Center in October 2013. I was just there a couple of days ago. The center is a premiere assembly of colleges devoted to educating health professionals and investigators through innovative teaching and research in dentistry, medicine, nursing, and biomedical sciences, and the list goes on and on. You served as vice chancellor for the Center of Innovation and Advanced Development. Your resume is very lengthy and very illustrative. Thank you for being here.

Next, we have the Honorable Clay Lewis Jenkins, county judge for Dallas County. He is responsible for the truancy court system. In addition, as the chief elected official of the county, Judge Jenkins is responsible for the county's disaster and emergency preparedness. He appointed a director of homeland security and emergency preparedness person to manage the county's 24-hour operation. Thank you for being here, sir.

Last, we have Dr. Troisi, who is an associate professor, Division of Management Policy and Community Health with the Center for Infectious Diseases at the University of Texas. She has expertise in infectious diseases, including influenza, hepatitis, sexually transmitted diseases, as well as outbreaks, including Ebola as well. Thank you so much for being here.

The Chairman now recognizes Dr. Lakey for his testimony.

STATEMENT OF DAVID LAKEY, M.D., COMMISSIONER OF HEALTH, TEXAS DEPARTMENT OF STATE HEALTH SERVICES

Dr. LAKEY. Good afternoon, and thank you, Chairman McCaul, and thank you, Ranking Member Sheila Jackson Lee, and thank you to all the Members that are here today. I thank you for this opportunity to discuss our efforts here in Dallas to prevent the spread of Ebola.

I want to start by saying that I know the people in Dallas and the rest of the State, and I know also in the rest of the Nation, are scared. Ebola is a frightening disease with grave health consequences. It is an unknown, something that we have never diagnosed here within the borders before, and the specter of the heartbreaking outbreak in West Africa reminds of how serious this situation could be.

But fortunately, Ebola is also a disease that we can fight through simple preventative public health measures, measures that we have in the United States and have long experience with, measures that have had success in that we can depend on their effectiveness.

Regretfully, as you know, Mr. Duncan lost his fight with Ebola on Wednesday, and my condolences really go out to the family right now. It is hard to image what he and his family have endured in the last 2 weeks, and the struggle for Mr. Duncan's family is not over yet. Our goal, however, is to minimize the possibility that other Texans will be exposed to Ebola and, thus, reduce the possibility of another case, another death, and another grieving family.

I know that for all of us our minds weigh heavy on the thought of Mr. Duncan's family right now and the 48 individuals and their loved ones who must wait another 2 weeks to feel confident in their health, uncertain of their future. As Texas State's health official, responsibility weighs heavy on me, that we identify every possible contact, that we take every precaution to prevent the spread of the disease, that we monitor individuals closely, and that we are earning the Texans' trust in public health prevention and control.

For decades, public health has taken the role of responding to infectious disease events. Public health response includes identification of individuals who have been exposed to a disease, monitoring people identified as having risk for exposure, and immediate care and public health follow-up should symptoms become apparent.

Every infectious disease event is different based on the nature of the disease and the scope of the event. Despite these differences, the response structure remains the same. In Texas, local authorities who best know their affected community lead response efforts. That is not to say, however, that local officials are alone in this response. Effective disease investigation also involves support by the State and by the Federal Government.

We at the Department of State Health Services are always prepared to offer local governments our knowledge and our experience as they respond to infectious disease events. When an event oustrips local capabilities, the State is ready as appropriate to take a leadership role. Similarly, the Centers for Disease Control and Prevention offers Federal expertise and advice, and can provide additional help for large-scale events and multi-jurisdictional events.

The norm in public health is for all three levels of government to work in tandem—local, State, and Federal government working together in what I call the public health enterprise, providing each other support and filling in gaps, to provide a cohesive response. I do want to take a second to thank the Centers for Disease Control for their on-going work here in the State of Texas, for their expertise, the help in our laboratory, the epidemiologists that are here in the State of Texas, here in Dallas right now.

This cooperative effort is not always easy, and it is not always executed perfectly, but this partnership will provide the best results and serve to best protect the public's health. In this particular incident, Dallas County Health and Human Services is the lead of the investigation and the response effort.

The Department of State Health Services and the Centers for Disease Control became very deeply involved early on given the significance of this deadly disease. In fact, our State laboratory at the Department of State Health Services recently qualified to test for Ebola in Austin and is one of 13 State laboratories able to do so. For this reason, we were involved very quickly, providing consultation about the possibility of testing and diagnosis and diagnosing the case in our laboratory.

As you know, we are still in the midst of this response. Forty-eight individuals are being monitored for symptoms of Ebola due to the risk of exposure. Ten of those individuals are considered high-risk. Our response won't be over until we can confidently rule out Ebola infection in each of these individuals. I want to reassure Texans and the folks in Dallas right now that none of these individuals are sick at this point, but keep in mind that the symptoms can become evident anywhere from 2 to 21 days after exposure.

As with all response efforts here in Texas, we are learning new lessons for improving our preparedness for outbreaks and for future disasters. At the end of each event, the Department of State Health Services immediately initiates an after-action review to determine what went well, what could be improved, and how those improvements should be made. The after-action process will include local, State, and Federal responders to ensure that we are looking at all aspects of this response.

In the mean time, two themes are apparent. First, we know that disease reporting systems work and is key to public health workers quickly stopping the spread of disease. Providers and facilities must be aware of the responsibility. We as an agency must do our part to reinforce this responsibility through reminders, through updates, and to easy-to-use reporting systems.

Second, providers must be aware of outbreaks world-wide so that they know what diagnoses are possible based on that very important travel history. Until the West Africa outbreak is over, Ebola must be in the differential diagnosis of those individuals who recently arrived from one of the outbreak countries. Again, as an agency we must do our part to remind providers and facilities about outbreaks in other countries through our current communication chains, by harnessing Federal reminders, and by keeping health care providers armed with up-to-date procedures and guidance.

The importance of taking a travel history cannot be understated given the interconnected world in which we live. After the Ebola response ends and there has been time to thoroughly evaluate the entire event, we will complete an analysis of the event in our plan to improve response efforts going forward.

In support of this effort and to improve the response in Texas, our Governor, Rick Perry, has announced the formation of the Texas Task Force for Infectious Disease Preparedness and Response to assist and enhance the State's capabilities to respond to outbreaks such as we are in right now. I am a member of this task force, and I look forward to working on this important effort with others who have expertise in fields like epidemiology, preparedness, and response.

For now, we are focusing on our immediate job, ensuring that there are no more exposures related to this case in Dallas. We know that we can complete this job successfully. We know this because the science is sound. Ebola spreads through the direct contact with bodily fluids, and there is very little risk otherwise. Individuals are not contagious until they have symptoms.

Ebola does not thrive in the environment, and it is easily killed. Infection control is prevalent in United States hospitals. We have the supplies, the equipment, and the protocols to minimize the chance of disease spread within our hospitals. Prevention in the community is simple: Maintaining hand-washing hygiene and to avoid direct contact with people who are medically suspected or known to have Ebola. Most importantly, we know that we can and will successfully complete this job because we have done so in the past.

The dependable results of sound public health measures have been proven on diseases like tuberculosis, measles, and Middle East Respiratory Syndrome. We have a history in public health of successfully containing the spread of disease and protecting the public, and I am confident we will do the same here with this case of Ebola. Thank you, sir.

[The prepared statement of Dr. Lakey follows:]

PREPARED STATEMENT OF DAVID LAKEY

On October 8, 2014, Thomas Eric Duncan passed away as a result of contracting the Ebola virus in Liberia. Mr. Duncan was provided therapeutic care at Texas Health Presbyterian Hospital in Dallas, Texas, but he was unfortunately unable to recover from this often fatal disease.

Mr. Duncan's death is a reminder of the importance of disease prevention and control, and provides additional meaning to efforts in Texas to prevent further exposure to the disease. The goal in Texas is to continue to minimize risk, thus reducing the likelihood of another Ebola death within the State.

Every sympathy and concern is extended to Mr. Duncan's family, as they both grieve for their loved one and worry for their own health.

BACKGROUND: EBOLA CASE IN DALLAS

On September 30, 2014, the Department of State Health Services (DSHS) Laboratory and Centers for Disease Control and Prevention (CDC) tested a specimen for Ebola virus, and found it positive. This is the first Ebola patient to be diagnosed in the country.

The patient contracted Ebola in Liberia, and was not symptomatic when travelling into the United States. Ebola is only communicable when an infected person is ill with symptoms. During the incubation period, when no symptoms are present, a person is not infectious.

Texas Presbyterian Hospital received the patient, and contacted the Dallas County Health and Human Services on September 28, 2014, after the patient was transported to the emergency room by ambulance. He had previously presented at the hospital on September 26, was evaluated, provided medications, and discharged. Dallas County contacted DSHS and the CDC, to allow for coordination. Texas Health and Safety Code, Chapter 81, requires that Viral Hemorrhagic Fever (Ebola) be immediately reported to the local health department, which in turn notifies State and Federal partners, as warranted.

Once Ebola was suspected as a possible diagnosis on the 28th, Dallas County began a public health investigation to determine if others were exposed to the virus while the patient was symptomatic. After the patient's diagnosis, DSHS and CDC staff were on-site to provide assistance in the epidemiological investigation. The initial investigation identified 114 individuals who may have had contact with the patient. Additional investigation narrowed this number down, and a total of 48 contacts of varying risk were identified for monitoring. The investigation is on-going.

Ebola symptoms can become evident between 2 and 21 days after the initial infection. However, 8 to 10 days is the most common time frame for Ebola symptoms to become apparent. Ebola is only transmittable through direct contact with blood or body fluid, or exposure through contaminated objects, such as needles. Direct contact requires exposure through broken skin or unprotected mucous membranes.

By determining whether contact with the patient occurred, and whether possible contact was direct or indirect, investigating epidemiologists concluded that 10 individuals should be considered high-risk exposures. All 48 identified contacts were placed under monitoring for symptoms, with regular visits from local, State, and CDC health department officials.

The 48 individuals will be monitored until they have passed the 21-day threshold for presentation of symptoms.

INFECTIOUS DISEASE SURVEILLANCE IN TEXAS

The State of Texas is divided into eight DSHS health service regions. In areas where a local health department exists, DSHS health service regional offices provide supplemental or supporting public health services. In areas where there is no local health department, DSHS health service regional offices act as the local health authority.

Local health departments are of varying size, resources, and capacities. While some health departments, like Dallas County, support a full array of services, others have more limited functions. Approximately 60 health departments in Texas are "full service," while 80 offer fewer services. DSHS' role is to fill in, as needed, core public health services not offered at the local level.

For infectious disease, DSHS health service regions ensure that disease surveillance occurs in every Texas county through the continual and systematic collection, analysis, and interpretation of health data. This effort is dependent on disease reporting by providers, which is required by law. Currently, in Texas, over 60 conditions are subject to mandatory reporting, including: Food-borne, vector-borne, respiratory, and sexually transmitted diseases. Viral Hemorrhagic Fever, or Ebola, is an immediately-reportable disease in Texas.

In order to allow real-time monitoring of disease surveillance data, the CDC provides and maintains the National Electronic Disease Surveillance Network (NEDSS) for use by local, regional, and State health departments. NEDSS is used by nearly every local health department in the State, and allows DSHS to identify unusual increases or pattern shifts in disease numbers.

In concert with NEDSS, Electronic Laboratory Reporting (ELR) has improved the timeliness and comprehensiveness of diseases reporting. ELR electronically links laboratory test reports to NEDSS, allowing immediate access by DSHS or the local health department with legal jurisdiction.

INFECTIOUS DISEASE INVESTIGATION AND RESPONSE IN TEXAS

Timely disease reporting to the public health system is imperative for quick mobilization of public health investigation and response efforts. Since Texas is a home-rule State, epidemiological investigations begin at the local level, unless there is no local health department. This local responsibility aids in effective epidemiological investigations by ensuring that investigations are based on close understanding of the community and its residents. While local entities have the statutory responsibility to lead infectious disease investigations, State and CDC guidance is available and widely-used.

More complicated or wide-spread events can increase the State and Federal roles. If an outbreak involves multiple jurisdictions, the State role becomes more prominent. If, at any time, an investigation goes beyond local capabilities, the State may take the lead. In turn, if an investigation exceeds State resources, the State may ask the CDC for assistance. Additionally, the CDC leads multi-State investigations. No matter the level of outbreak, the norm is for all three levels of Government to work in cooperation, with varying levels of State and Federal involvement depending on the size and type of infectious disease event, and the resources and expertise of the local entity. Throughout the event in Dallas, the State and local authorities have been supported by CDC, both in the field and by home office staff.

Support provided by the State and CDC can include a number of options, depending on the scope of an investigation and local needs. This support might consist of subject-matter expertise and on-site assistance; State or CDC laboratory testing; provision of personal protection equipment; or mobilizing of DSHS Rapid Assessment Teams or CDC Epi-Aids. The State and CDC can also assist with administering questionnaires and interviews to cases and potential contacts, inspecting relevant hospital facilities or restaurants, and helping examine pertinent records.

In cases of large-scale outbreaks, the State Medical Operations Center (SMOC) at DSHS may be activated. The SMOC is staffed by DSHS Community Preparedness, Infectious Disease, and Communications staff. Its function is to ease the flow of information among multiple jurisdictions, provide dependable tracking of events, and facilitate requests for resources and supplies from local jurisdictions. For the Ebola case and investigation in Dallas, the SMOC has been activated.

SUCCESSFUL INFECTIOUS DISEASE RESPONSE IN TEXAS

The public health response system in Texas, led by local entities and supported by State and Federal government, has a long history of successful outbreak responses. Texas has effectively contained events involving disease like Tuberculosis, measles, hepatitis, and Middle East Respiratory Syndrome (MERS).

As an example, DSHS disease investigators are currently assisting the local health authority in El Paso, Texas, to track a number of exposures to Tuberculosis (TB) that occurred through a health care worker in the labor and delivery unit of a local hospital. This situation is a prime example of how, under the current system, all levels of government successfully work together to respond to an infectious disease event.

Once the index case was identified, local and State health department investigators meticulously examined hospital records to determine infants, parents, coworkers, and volunteers who were at risk of exposure. This investigation identified an initial 3,227 potentially-exposed newborns, and 69 potentially-exposed health care workers. Together, public health workers evaluated the index case's history to determine where exposure may have actually occurred. Then, they prioritized potential contacts by level of risk, decided on a contact investigation protocol specific to this incident, and executed the contact investigation. The CDC has been on-site to provide assistance, and home office CDC staff has provided expertise and advice. International coordination took place due to the city's proximity to the U.S.-Mexico Border; interstate coordination with New Mexico was also necessary.

While the investigation is not yet complete, its results are already evident. Public health investigators were able to narrow down the initial 3,227 number to 757 infants who had some level of risk of exposure. Follow-up with parents occurred, and testing was recommended, as appropriate, for potentially-exposed children. Additionally, DSHS gave providers guidance on treatment algorithms for possible cases. Of the 503 infants tested, six have tested positive for TB infection, and are being treated to ensure they do not develop active TB. Of the 58 health care workers tested, four tested positive for TB infection, and public health follow-up will ensure that these positive cases do not develop into a risk for further community exposure.

INITIAL LESSONS LEARNED: EBOLA CASE AND INVESTIGATION IN DALLAS, TEXAS

The Ebola investigation is on-going, but events like the TB exposure in El Paso and past infectious disease events reveal key themes to successful prevention and control of disease outbreaks in Texas and in the country.

The crux of infectious disease response is reporting. Providers must be aware of what diseases are reportable to their local health department, and promptly report contagious disease through the reporting system. Provider awareness of this responsibility allows for more effective disease surveillance, and more timely response to developing infectious disease events. DSHS works to reinforce this requirement through reminders, updates, and by making the reporting system user-friendly.

Secondly, the Ebola case in Dallas highlights the need for providers to vigilantly take travel histories, and streamline sharing of this information while a patient is being diagnosed. Providers must be aware of outbreaks worldwide, to inform their consideration of patient travel history. Until the Ebola outbreak in West Africa is over, Ebola must be a differential diagnosis for those who have recently traveled from one of the outbreak countries. At the same time, moving forward, providers must be aware of what other outbreaks are occurring internationally. Electronic notifications from the CDC help providers stay informed, and these messages can be strengthened through State and local-level communications.

AFTER-ACTION ASSESSMENTS

After the response to the Ebola case and investigation comes to a close, DSHS will perform an after-action review of the response to this situation. Throughout the event, responders keep in mind how the response flows, what difficulties are encountered, and what successes are achieved. After the response, a thoughtful assessment brings all these experiences into one evaluation. An after-action review is essential to close out any response effort, in order to improve future responses. The assessment will include input from local, State, and Federal responders who were part of the effort, and will analyze each part of the response. The assessment will determine what worked, what can be improved, and how those improvements can be made. The final result will be enhanced preparedness plans for future infectious disease events.

In addition, Texas Governor Rick Perry has formed a Texas Task Force on Infectious Disease Preparedness and Response, the purpose of which is to assess and enhance the State's capabilities to respond to outbreak situations. The task force is composed of 17 members, headed by infectious disease and Ebola experts, and will be supported by DSHS and other State agencies. The Task Force will evaluate infectious disease response in Texas, and determine what recommendations can be made for improvements, either through agency or legislative action. The Task Force will make its report to the Texas State Legislature in December 2014.

CONCLUSION

The response to the Ebola case in Dallas is on-going. Conclusion of this event will allow a systematic review of the response efforts, and the Governor's Task Force on

Infectious Disease Preparedness and Response will facilitate an evaluation of the public health response system as a whole. It is evident from a long history of success that public health interventions work, and that infectious disease investigation and follow-up can stop the spread of disease. However, each infectious disease event provides a new opportunity to make improvements to disease investigation response and coordination among public health entities. The current focus is on ensuring that no more Texans are exposed to the Ebola virus. When that mission is complete, the focus will shift to recommending and implementing improved plans for future infectious disease response in Texas.

Chairman McCAUL. Thank you, Dr. Lakey.

The Chairman recognizes Dr. Giroir.

STATEMENT OF BRETT P. GIROIR, M.D., EXECUTIVE VICE PRESIDENT AND CEO, TEXAS A&M HEALTH SCIENCE CENTER, AND DIRECTOR, TEXAS TASK FORCE ON INFECTIOUS DISEASE PREPAREDNESS AND RESPONSE

Dr. GIROIR. Mr. Chairman, Members of the committee, thank you for inviting me to testify before you today. By training I am a critical care physician and formerly served in the Federal Government as director of the Science Office at DARPA and also on the Defense Threat Reduction Advisory Committee where I chaired the biological and chemical panel.

On Monday, October 6, Governor Perry named me as the director of the Texas Task Force on Infectious Disease Preparedness and Response. The task force includes internationally-recognized biomedical experts joined by State agency CEOs, not only from Health and Human Services, but also from transportation, environmental regulation, public education, and diverse other areas.

Why such diversity? Because the Dallas case proves that an effective response requires much more than public health professionals alone. For example, waste disposal was complicated by broad challenges, including decontamination decisions, temporary housing, availability of containers, vehicle logistics and availabilities, and permitting for transportation and disposal spanning multiple jurisdictions. Cleaning a single apartment generated 140 55-gallon containers of Class A hazardous waste, each of which then needed to be transported to an incinerator licensed for such disposal.

We believe that the response and coordination of local, State, and Federal resources in Dallas has been very good, but there will be areas for improvement and lessons learned. Our task force has already been very active and has identified seven major areas for assessment and recommendation. These include hospital preparedness for patient identification and isolation; command and control, including education and activation of the incident command structures, implementation of epidemiological investigations and patient monitoring; decontamination and waste disposal; complexities of patient care, including use of experimental therapies; care of contacts being monitored by public health officials; and as highlighted in the Spanish case, we have also added management of domestic animal exposures.

Now, I would like to respectfully offer three suggestions for consideration by Congress and the President on how to improve our preparedness and response. The first is to reestablish the special assistant to the President for biodefense. Doing so would restore leadership, accountability, and consistent prioritization at the highest level of Government. This position had existed both under the President Clinton and President Bush administrations, and I would refer you to Congressman Thornberry and Congressman Langeven's letter to the President on April 22, 2014 about this very subject.

Point No. 2, restore funding to hospital preparedness programs. Our Nation's public health infrastructure has been significantly impeded by cuts to the Federal Hospital Preparedness Program, which has been reduced from approximately $500 million per year in fiscal year 2007 and 2008 to $230 million today. There should also, however, be clear metrics for success, accountability for that success, and close integration with FEMA emergency management programs.

Point No. 3, set clear deliverables and accountability for new vaccines and therapies. In terms of the availability of medical countermeasures against Ebola and many other threats, our country is woefully deficient. This relates both to scientific and technical obstacles, but also a lack of prioritization, accountability, and funding that is based on outcomes. As the Government is now prioritizing Ebola, it is critical that we backfill all funding that has been redirected from other biodefense priorities. We should not fight the battle against Ebola at the cost of forfeiting the broader war against other menacing diseases, such as pandemic influenza or Middle Eastern Respiratory Syndrome.

On a final note is that the Texas A&M Health Science Center is home to one of three BARTA-funded National centers to develop and manufacture vaccines and medical countermeasures against chemical, biological, radiological, and nuclear threats. Each center, including our own, will be responsible for producing 50 million pandemic vaccine doses within 4 months of receipt of the referenced strain. Our center and the others are also fully capable of supporting development and manufacture of vaccines and therapeutics against Ebola if requested by the Federal Government.

In closing, thank you, Chairman McCaul, and the Members of the committee for your leadership and for engaging on this critical aspect of National security.

[The prepared statement of Dr. Giroir follows:]

PREPARED STATEMENT OF BRETT P. GIROIR

Chairman McCaul and Members of the committee: I am Dr. Brett Giroir, chief executive officer of Texas A&M Health Science Center, and professor in the Colleges of Medicine and Engineering. By training, I am a critical care physician-scientist with specific experience in treating life-threatening infectious diseases. I also have experience in the Federal Government as director of the Defense Sciences Office at the Defense Advanced Research Projects Agency (DARPA) and chair of the Chemical and Biological Defense Panel of the Department of Defense Threat Reduction Advisory Committee. In addition, earlier this week, Governor Perry named me director of the Texas Task Force on Infectious Disease Preparedness and Response.

The risk of infectious disease outbreaks is real, and these outbreaks are inevitable given the interconnected nature of the world we live in. An outbreak anywhere becomes a threat everywhere. Given our location along the U.S. border, our experience with major natural disasters, and our unique assets such as the Galveston National Laboratory and the Texas A&M Center for Innovation in Advanced Development and Manufacturing (CIADM), Texas is on the front lines of public health preparedness and protection.

In response to the first case of Ebola diagnosed in the United States, Governor Perry swiftly established the Task Force on Infectious Disease Preparedness and

Response to assess and manage the risk in Texas and to prospectively plan for future infectious disease threats—whether natural or the result of bioterrorist attacks. The Task Force includes internationally-recognized infectious disease and public health experts, seasoned biodefense leaders, and State agency professionals across major areas including health and human services, emergency management, public safety, transportation, environmental quality, public education, and housing and community affairs. The members of this task force volunteered in order to serve the people of Texas, and as a result, the Nation, and each of us has accepted this call to duty from the Governor for that sole purpose.

There is no question that there will be opportunities for increased performance across many of the complex elements that have been brought together to effectively contain Ebola within Texas. Remember, this was the first Ebola patient to be diagnosed in the United States. If there is room for improvement, we will work to assure that Texas learns, documents, disseminates information, and implements optimal changes to further protect our citizens—and that the United States, as a whole, benefits from the process. The Texas Task Force took action right away, meeting for the first time immediately after the Governor issued the executive order, and we have been actively engaged in assessments and discussion since that time. We have preliminarily identified six areas of focus that have been prominent in the current Ebola response, and we believe that these areas will have implications for many potential disease outbreaks should they arrive in the United States. These areas include:

1. *Hospital Preparedness and the Potential Role of Improved Rapid Diagnostics.*—The Task Force will focus on the initial identification of a patient, or potential patient, and the education and preparedness of diverse health care professionals essential for this key step in the containment process.

2. *Command and Control Issues.*—The Task Force will focus on processes related to the initial activation of the Incident Command Structure, integration of local, State, and Federal resources, development of a common operating picture, and the unique differences of a public health challenge, such as an Ebola patient, compared to the challenges experienced in natural disasters such as hurricanes.

3. *Organization and Implementation of Epidemiologic Investigations and Monitoring.*—The Task Force will assess opportunities for improved integration of disease tracking, data and information synthesis, and potential opportunities for automated technologies and scalable common data platforms that could be shared at the local, State, and Federal levels.

4. *Decontamination and Waste Disposal.*—The Task Force will review and assess a plethora of issues faced in this area, including but not limited to: Determining what could be decontaminated, versus contained-hauled-incinerated, availability of appropriate containers, logistics of transport, and complex permitting issues across multiple levels of jurisdiction.

5. *Patient Care Issues.*—The Task Force will examine how to improve information flow to front-line care providers, including information on new drugs, their risks and potential benefits, and how they might be accessed under investigational protocols.

6. *Care of Patients Being Monitored.*—The Task Force will examine the diverse needs of individuals under monitoring or controlled monitoring, including the needs for basic necessities, such as food, clothing, and housing, as well as potential needs for social services and/or counseling. Due to the rich diversity of the Texas population, cultural competency in communication and interactions are important aspects of this area.

The Task Force will submit initial draft assessments and recommendations by December 1 for consideration by the Office of the Governor and Texas Legislature, so that actions requiring statutory changes could be proposed in the 2015 legislative session. In the mean time, the Task Force is committed to insuring that the teams on the ground have all necessary expertise and resources at their disposal to respond to the potential for additional Ebola cases in Texas, and to begin the process of developing an infectious disease preparedness and response plan to complement the State Emergency Management Plan already in place and proven highly effective in response to natural disasters.

Regarding the current situation here in Dallas, the response and coordination of local, State, and Federal resources has generally been very good, but the Task Force will seek opportunities for improvement at all levels of collaboration and integration. Looking forward, the issues at hand are highly dependent on the larger security and preparedness system. State and local planning is critical, but so is clear and defined support to local and State authorities from the Federal Government, including the Centers for Disease Control (CDC) and Office of the Assistant Secretary for Preparedness and Response (ASPR). While there have been lessons learned, the successes in controlling this potentially dangerous situation are a testament to the incredible skill and dedication of all those on the ground in Dallas, who in my mind are nothing less than National heroes.

GAPS IN HOSPITAL PREPAREDNESS AND PUBLIC HEALTH INFRASTRUCTURE

It is important to understand that our State's and the Nation's public health infrastructure has been subject to significant funding reductions in the Federal Hospital Preparedness Program (HPP), which is intended to provide funding and support to improve surge capacity and enhance community and hospital preparedness for public health emergencies. These funds are expressly for enhanced planning at the State and local level, for increased integration across the public and private health care sectors, including hospitals, and other health care organizations and providers, and for improving infrastructure for public health emergencies. It should come as no surprise that hospitals require public funding to train and prepare for what are low-probability yet high-consequence, and potentially catastrophic, events.

HPP is meant to provide the foundation and core for exercises and ability to respond and get information out so that the nurse or physician on the front line would contemplate Ebola or anthrax in their differential diagnosis. HPP has been cut significantly in recent years by the Federal Government, and these actions have had clear, identifiable consequences here in Dallas. In fact, during the Federal Budget compromise last year, HPP funds were diverted to fund the Biomedical Advanced Research and Development Authority (BARDA) rather than use another funding source that was suggested by Congressional leaders. While we are very thankful this action allowed BARDA to continue operations (especially since the importance of its mission has been made abundantly clear during this Ebola response) robbing Peter to pay Paul has left us less far less prepared than we could have been, and indeed should have been. This must change if we are to be prepared for public health emergencies, now and in the future.

GUIDELINES FOR HEALTH PREPAREDNESS AND TECHNOLOGICAL FIELD SUPPORT

In January 2012, ASPR issued "Healthcare Preparedness Capabilities," providing National guidelines for health care system preparedness. Unfortunately, several of the critical capabilities identified in the report remain problematic areas in our public health preparedness and response infrastructure.

For instance, ASPR recommendations address the ability to coordinate multiple agencies and their decision making, to provide incident information sharing, to manage resource implementation, to provide an inventory management system, and to notify stakeholders of health care delivery status. In reality, the incident command team does not have the necessary technology in place to provide data tracking and analysis that would support the prescribed common operating picture across the multiple layers necessary to coordinate an effective and integrated response. Currently, information is housed on individual laptops and other devices, being reported manually, and compiled once or twice daily for the Texas Department of State Health Services Commissioner, Dr. David Lakey, who is leading the response in Dallas, and to whom we all owe a debt of gratitude, along with his colleagues in the CDC and other responders, who are working around these technological coordination challenges to the degree possible.

Another critical capability outlined by the ASPR report, Information Sharing, is to "Provide health care situational awareness that contributes to the incident common operating picture." This critical capability has not been realized in the current Ebola scenario. In short, our public health infrastructure has not kept pace with technological and communications breakthroughs that are now wide-spread, and also has not yet incorporated tools to facilitate data collection, analysis, communication, and decision making. This reality must be acknowledged by ASPR leadership, and a strategy to address these significant challenges should be developed in partnership with the caregivers at the epicenter of the current Ebola containment mission.

NATIONAL INVENTORY OF POTENTIALLY AVAILABLE EBOLA THERAPEUTICS

Another major gap is the lack of any sort of inventory of candidate therapeutics to treat Ebola patients who are brought to the United States for treatment or who are diagnosed in our country. The fact of the matter is that we had a person fighting for his life on American soil and no easily available information about drugs available to administer. This is not a new issue; Dr. Keith Brantley received ZMapp in August by hearing about it from a colleague, not from U.S. Federal authorities. Unfortunately, because of a number of issues as further described in this testimony, ZMapp was not available to be given to Mr. Duncan.

The Federal Government should provide a timely and frequently-updated list of all possible medical countermeasures to treating physicians or to appropriate State public health officials. This list should include a concise summary of risks and potential benefits, instructions for how to obtain these therapies, and also should insure that there are specific research protocols in place to capture the meaningful data that will be generated through the use of these drugs. Today, physicians and patients often must track down the companies directly and ask for the drug candidates, or officials such as myself use personal contacts within the Government to provide as much information as possible to the hospital treatment team. This is both inefficient and time-consuming—and thus leaves patients and doctors less than optimally equipped in this struggle for life and death of a critically-ill patient. This is completely unacceptable given the more than decade-long effort the Federal Government has undertaken to evaluate and advance medical countermeasures.

In terms of availability of therapies or vaccines against Ebola, our country is woefully and indeed frighteningly deficient. While it is true that the mainstay of Ebola treatment is supportive care, that is only the case because we have little else to offer. It is my personal assessment after experiences in both the academic and Federal sectors that this deficiency relates less to scientific and technical obstacles, than it does to the lack of Federal prioritization of the efforts; lack of clear Federal leadership accountability; and difficult, if not oppressive, contracting procedures that are often at odds with the iterated National strategy and objectives.

SPECIAL ASSISTANT TO THE PRESIDENT ON BIODEFENSE

When Congress created the assistant secretary for preparedness and response role in 2006 as part of the Pandemics and All Hazards Preparedness Act, ASPR was intended precisely for the kind of situation we face today with Ebola. The Nation was to be provided with a Senate-confirmed assistant secretary to take an all-hazards approach to bring to bear all necessary resources, regardless of where they belong on the Federal Government's organizational chart. That resource exists today in ASPR, but what is critically lacking is a White House Special Assistant to prepare for and lead such responses. Unfortunately, that position was eliminated by the current administration in January 2009.

We commend Chairman W. "Mac" Thornberry and James Langevin, Ranking Member, of the House Armed Services Committee Subcommittee on Intelligence, Emerging Threats, and Capabilities, for their April 22, 2014 letter to the President on this very topic, in which they call for the appointment of a Special Assistant to the President for Biodefense. This position has existed under both the Clinton and Bush administrations but was eliminated early in 2009. The letter notes that "there are at least 12 separate Government agencies with biodefense responsibilities." As pointed out in a 2001 U.S. Government Accountability Office report, "Opportunities to Reduce Potential Duplication in Government Programs, Save Tax Dollars, and Enhance Revenue," there are more than "two dozen Presidentially-appointed individuals with some responsibility for biodefense."

CONTRACTING AUTHORITY

ASPR, which is housed within the U.S. Department of Health and Human Services, oversees BARDA and the Office of Acquisitions Management, Contracts and Grants (AMCG). Several years ago an administrative decision was made to centralize all contracting under AMCG, and remove it from under BARDA's responsibility. While this made sense at the time, in practice, this has significantly slowed BARDA's efforts to move medical countermeasures through the manufacturing pipeline. Returning contracting authority to BARDA would certainly clear the way for the development of medical countermeasures, including experimental Ebola therapies. I want to specifically state that my team, and indeed most if not all of the scientific and technical community, has great respect for the leadership and technical expertise of BARDA. Without BARDA, the country would be gravely behind the curve without even the basic National response infrastructure to address this problem, or ever-present global challenges such as pandemic influenza.

TEXAS A&M CIADM AND EBOLA THERAPEUTICS

As you know, the Texas A&M Center for Innovation in Advanced Development and Manufacturing is a public-public-private partnership with the U.S. Department of Health and Human Services and 1 of 3 Government-funded biosecurity centers designed to enhance the Nation's preparedness against pandemic influenza, and chemical, biological, radiological, and nuclear threats by accelerating the research and development of vaccines and therapeutics, and rapidly manufacturing these products at scale in cases of National emergencies. The Texas A&M CIADM is responsible for producing 50 million vaccine doses within 4 months of a declared influenza pandemic and receipt of the viral strain. It is also responsible for having the capabilities to manufacture, at scale, vaccines or biological therapeutics required for an outbreak, such as Ebola, if requested by the Federal Government. Our team is made up of leading academic, non-profit, and commercial partners including GSK.

The Texas A&M CIADM represents a long-term, strategic initiative—sponsored by BARDA—to assure preparedness by creating indispensable infrastructure and staff capabilities to rapidly respond against highly diverse threats. The CIADM will deliver on several critical objectives, including:

- Ensure the United States can develop and manufacture life-saving vaccines and therapies quickly, flexibly, and cost effectively at scale;
- Improve the ability to protect the health of Americans in response to emergency situations; and
- Train an expert workforce that can fill the needs of National biosecurity for the next generation.

The Center stands ready, and if called upon, will compete for manufacturing of a wide range of vaccines or therapeutics required by the U.S. Government, including products against Ebola. Texas A&M Health Science Center also has a proprietary vaccine candidate now in preclinical evaluation that holds promise as one of the weapons against this growing global threat.

In closing, I thank you Chairman McCaul, and the Members of the committee for your leadership and for engaging on this important series of challenges that I have outlined. The members of the Texas Task Force and Texas A&M Center for Innovation want to be seen as your partners in solving the current Ebola situation in Texas and building a resilient and prepared homeland that can overcome threats, regardless of the source. I am honored and privileged to serve as resource to you now and going forward.

Chairman MCCAUL. Thank you, Dr. Giroir. Let me say the Governor, I believe, made an excellent choice appointing you to be the head of this task force. Thank you.

Dr. GIROIR. Thank you, sir.

Chairman MCCAUL. Judge Jenkins.

STATEMENT OF HON. CLAY LEWIS JENKINS, JUDGE, DALLAS COUNTY, TEXAS

Judge JENKINS. Well, thank you, Chairman McCaul, Congresswoman Sheila Jackson Lee, Members of this committee, and my friends from the Texas delegation who are here with us today. Thank you for your support in this challenging response.

Local government has treated everyone involved in the Ebola with dignity, and compassion, and as fellow human beings, not merely as disease contacts. In interacting with Louise and those three young men, it was important that I followed all CDC protocols to avoid any chance of spreading that virus. But it was important that I not move that family wearing a hazmat suit. It was important for them to see me as a fellow human being face-to-face, and for me to converse with them as equals. That is a basic tenant of leadership, and it is in keeping with modern medicine.

Louise Troh and those three young men have been handling an extraordinarily scary, sad, and difficult situation with grace. Louise and Eric's 19-year-old son, Karsiah, is a fine young man, forced to deal with the loss of his father without being able to hug and hold his mother. The death of Eric Duncan is the loss of a father, a fiancé, a son, and a person that was loved by an extended family.

Forty-eight people were found to be potentially exposed, disease contacts, by the excellent epidemiological and disease detection work performed by Dallas County, the State of Texas, and the Federal Government. For these 48 people and their families, this remains a tense and anxious period. They all need our thoughts and prayers, thankfully all without symptoms or fever on this the 12th day of monitoring.

We are one team, one fight, and we are committed to working together. We activated our Dallas County Emergency Operations Center, and we are operating under the incident command system with Federal, State, county, and city assets. Many partners, but one team, one team and one fight. Simply put, there is no other way to stop Ebola.

There is a lot of fear out there, and I understand why. Ebola is a scary, terrible disease. However, there is a 0 percent chance of contracting Ebola without coming into contact with the bodily fluids of a symptomatic Ebola victim. People who have been exposed to Ebola but have no fever or symptoms cannot transmit the virus.

We must not allow fear and panic to weaken our resolve, nor force us to abandon the values that that have built this great country. Everybody has a job to do in this outbreak. The Federal, State, and local governments are doing their job. I urge Congress to pass the appropriations necessary to fight Ebola in Africa, which is the best way to stem the epidemic, protect humankind, and for you to perform your important role in the strengthening and streamlining of Ebola response in the United States.

We are doing something that has not been done before, and we cannot fail. We will contain Ebola in Dallas, Texas. It is only a matter of time before the next case comes to our shores. Help us win this fight. We must win now. Work with us to fight this disease abroad and strengthen our public health security. Thank you.

[The prepared statement of Judge Jenkins follows:]

PREPARED STATEMENT OF CLAY LEWIS JENKINS

OCTOBER 10, 2014

Local government has treated everyone involved in this Ebola crisis with dignity and compassion as fellow human beings; not merely as disease contacts.

In interacting with the family, it was important that I followed all CDC protocols to avoid any chance of spreading the virus. It was also important that I not move the family while wearing a hazmat suit; for them to see me face-to-face and for me to converse with them as equals.

That is a basic tenet of leadership and in keeping with modern medicine.

Louise Troh and the three young men have been handling an extraordinarily scary, sad, and difficult situation with grace. Louise and Eric's 19-year-old son Karsiah is a fine young man forced to deal with the loss of his father without being able to hug and hold his mother.

The death of Eric Duncan is the loss of a father, fiancée, son, and person loved by an extended family.

Forty-eight people were found to be potentially-exposed disease contacts by the excellent epidemiological and disease-detection work performed by Dallas County, the State of Texas and the Federal Government. For these 48 people and their families, this remains a tense and anxious period. They need all of our thoughts and prayers. Thankfully, all are without symptoms or fever on this twelfth day of monitoring.

We are one team, one fight, and we are committed to working together.

We activated our Dallas County Emergency Operations Center and are operating under the Incident Command System with Federal, State, county, and city assets. Many partners, but one team.

One Team, One Fight! Simply said, there is no other way to stop Ebola.

There is a lot of fear out there and I understand why. Ebola is a scary, terrible viral disease. However, there is a 0 percent chance of contracting Ebola without coming into contact with the bodily fluids of a symptomatic Ebola victim. People who have been exposed to Ebola but have no fever or symptoms cannot transmit the virus. We must not allow fear and panic to weaken our resolve nor abandon the values that built this great Nation.

Everybody has a job to do in this outbreak. The Federal, State, and local governments are doing their jobs. I urge Congress to pass the appropriations necessary to fight Ebola in Africa which is the best way to stem the epidemic, protect humankind, and for you to perform your important role in strengthening and streamlining the Ebola response in the United States.

We are doing something that has not been done before and we cannot fail. We will contain Ebola in Dallas, Texas. It's only a matter of time before the next case comes to our shores. Help us, help us win this fight. We must win now. Work with us to fight this disease abroad and strengthen our public health security.

Chairman MCCAUL. Thank you, Judge.

The Chairman recognizes Dr. Troisi.

STATEMENT OF CATHERINE L. TROISI, PH.D., ASSOCIATE PROFESSOR, DIVISION OF MANAGEMENT, POLICY, AND COMMUNITY HEALTH CENTER FOR INFECTIOUS DISEASES, THE UNIVERSITY OF TEXAS

Ms. TROISI. Thank you. Chairman McCaul, Ranking Member Jackson Lee, and Members of the committee, I am Catherine Troisi, an infectious disease epidemiologist at the University of Texas School of Public Health, and I have also practiced public health at the local level. I am a member of the American Public Health Association and the Texas Public Health Association. Adequate funding of all levels of public health system is a top priority for these organizations.

I would like to start with a definition of "public health," a term that is sometimes confused with "medical care." "Public health" is defined as "all organized measures to prevent disease, promote health, and prolong life among the population as a whole." While medical care is concerned with the individual, public health's patient is the community.

I would argue that this definition of "public health" puts it in the realm of public safety. Just as police and firefighters protect communities from crime and blazes, public health protects communities from disease. Indeed, of the 30 years of added life to the U.S. life expectancy during the last century, 25 of these are due not to medical advances, but to public health interventions, such as sanitation, immunizations, workforce safety, tobacco control, et cetera. It has been said that health care is vital to all of us some of the time, but public health is vital to all of us all of the time.

I hope that I have convinced you of the importance of public health efforts in maintaining and promoting the health of our Nation and the world. This cannot be done without adequate resources. I am sure that you are much more familiar than I with the negative effects of spending caps and sequestration on public health agencies, such as the CDC. Federal funding for public health has declined in recent years, and this has affected flow-through funding to States and locals. Adjusted for inflation, CDC funding has decreased more than $1 billion since 2005, 15 percent.

At the State level, the Association of State and Territorial Health Officials reports that budget cuts continue to affect the health of Americans. Health departments in 48 States have had budgets cut since 2008, with 95 percent of departments reducing services that they offer. The Trust for America's Health and the RWJ Foundation released a report showing that the majority of States reached only half or fewer of key indicators of policies and capabilities to protect against infectious disease threats. Texas scored 4 out of 10. One of the indicators, increased or maintained level of funding, was not met by 33 States.

The same trends can be found at the local level. The National Association of County and City Health Officials reported that over one-quarter of local health departments experienced a budget cut in the current fiscal year, and this has been happening over at least the last 6 years. Almost half of these had reductions in services. Overall, State and local public health departments, the boots-on-the-ground providers of public health, have lost over 51,000 jobs since 2008. This represents 20 percent of public health jobs at the State and local level.

Ebola is a frightening disease with horrific symptoms, and concern is naturally high that spread may occur in the United States. However, this is highly unlikely. To be infected, you must have physical contact with bodily fluids from someone with symptoms. We know how to stop transmission by using barrier nursing practices, such as gloves, disinfectants, and patient isolation.

Unfortunately, many countries in Africa do not have the resources to provide for these precautions. Ebola is a major concern for the affected countries, and the fear and loss of life are devastating on a humanitarian level. The danger is that we will be fixated on this virus and not on other pathogens that have outbreak potential, such as flu, SARS, and MERS-CoV, among others. Other pathogens, such as measles and pertussis, periodically cause outbreaks due to lack of immunity among those not vaccinated. Then there is the on-going syphilis, food-borne illnesses, HIV, tuberculosis, meningitis, enterovirus D68 infections that we fight every day in public health.

So what can we do to prepare for potential pandemics? Congress must begin to prioritize public health funding and not just when a crisis occurs. Critical to the capacity to respond to any type of outbreak, routine or otherwise, are epidemiologic and laboratory capabilities. These involve disease surveillance and reporting, case investigation, outbreak response and control, contact management, and data analysis synthesis and communication.

The disease-of-the-month type of response limits our ability to react to threats, and disease-specific funding streams tie public health hands when prioritizing activities. While we are appreciative of the increased funding to combat Ebola, and adequate response to the initial outbreak would have mitigated spread. The U.S. funding for WHO activities have decreased one-third from 2010 to 2013.

In summary, public health is on a par with police and fire protecting the community from disease. In order to provide this protection, we need on-going adequate funding to make sure our epidemiologists and laboratories have the resources they need to quickly identify and stop infectious disease outbreaks.

Thank you for the opportunity to testify about public health and our ability to deal with public health threats.

[The prepared statement of Ms. Troisi follows:]

PREPARED STATEMENT OF CATHERINE L. TROISI

OCTOBER 10, 2014

Chairman McCaul, Ranking Member Thompson, and Members of the committee, my name is Catherine Troisi. I am an infectious disease epidemiologist at the University of Texas School of Public Health and, in addition to my years in academia, I have practiced public health at the Houston Department of Health and Human Services. I am also a member of the American Public Health Association, a diverse community of public health professionals who champion the health of all people and communities. Adequate funding at all levels of our public health system is a top priority for the association

Thank you for this opportunity to talk about public health, its role in disease outbreak detection, and recent trends in resources for these important public safety efforts. I'm delighted to remind the Members from Texas that the University of Texas School of Public Health has regional campuses in Austin, Brownsville, Dallas, El Paso, and San Antonio, fulfilling our mission to improve and sustain the health of people by providing the highest quality graduate education, research, and community service for Texas, the Nation, and the world; to provide quality graduate education in the basic disciplines and practices of public health; to extend the evidence base within those disciplines; and to assist public health practitioners, locally, Nationally, and internationally, in solving public health problems.

I'd like to start with a definition of public health, a term that is sometimes confused with medical care. Public health has been defined by the U.S. Centers for Disease Control and Prevention (CDC, the Nation's public health agency) as "the science of protecting and improving the health of families and communities through promotion of healthy lifestyles, research for disease and injury prevention and detection and control of infectious diseases." There are a couple of concepts in that definition I'd like to emphasize. The first is that public health is science-based and the corollary of that is that we should employ techniques that have been proven to be of value. The second is the idea of protection which implies action before disease occurs. Public health has two main functions—disease prevention and health promotion. As our grandmothers said "an ounce of prevention is worth a pound of cure". The last concept in this definition that I want to emphasize is that of communities. While traditional medical care is concerned with the individual, public health's "patient" is the community. Individual interventions can be the mandate of public health, e.g., immunizations, but the overall goal is to protect the community. One specific function of public health agencies, largely limited to governmental public health, is detection of outbreaks of infectious diseases and mitigation of spread.

With these definitions in mind, what are public health tasks? The Institute of Medicine has broken these into three core functions—assessment, policy development, and assurance. In simple terms, this means that public health is responsible for evaluating and responding to health problems in the community as well as prioritizing these efforts, developing policies to protect communities' health, and assuring that all populations have access to appropriate and cost-effective prevention services. I would argue that this academic and functional definition of public health puts it in the realm of public safety. Just as police protect communities from crime and fire fighters from the devastations of fire, public health protects communities from disease. Indeed, of the 30 years of life expectancy added to the average U.S. life expectancy in the 20th Century, 25 of these are due, not to medical care, but to public health interventions, such as sanitation, immunizations, control of infectious diseases, tobacco control, etc. It's important to emphasize that we talk about the "public health system" which consists of all organizations involved in protecting and improving the health of the community, whether Governmental, medical, non-profit, educational, social services, etc. However, given the scope of these hearings and the fact that it is Governmental public health that is largely concerned with detecting and controlling infectious disease outbreaks, I'm going to be talking about governmental local, State, and National public health.

I hope that I have convinced you of the importance of public health efforts in maintaining and promoting the health of our Nation and our world. Obviously, this cannot be done without adequate resources. Public health activities occur at the Federal, State, and local level and are funded as such. However, the CDC and other Federal agencies provide flow through funding for many public health activities at the State and local level. I'm sure that you are much more familiar than I with the negative effects of spending caps and sequestration on public health agencies such as the CDC over the past few years. However, in a nutshell, Federal funding for public health has been relatively flat-funded and has shown a significant decline in recent years (Figure 1).

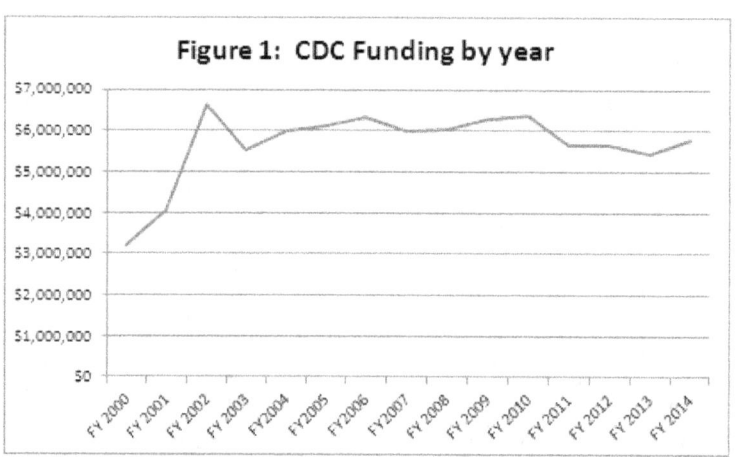

Figure 1: CDC Funding by year

Figure 2 shows the declining level of terrorism preparedness and emergency response funding allotted to CDC for activities at the National, State, and local levels and for the Strategic National Stockpile (*www.cdc.gov/fmo/topic/Budget%20Information/index.html*). Following infusion of after 9/11, levels have been on the decline.

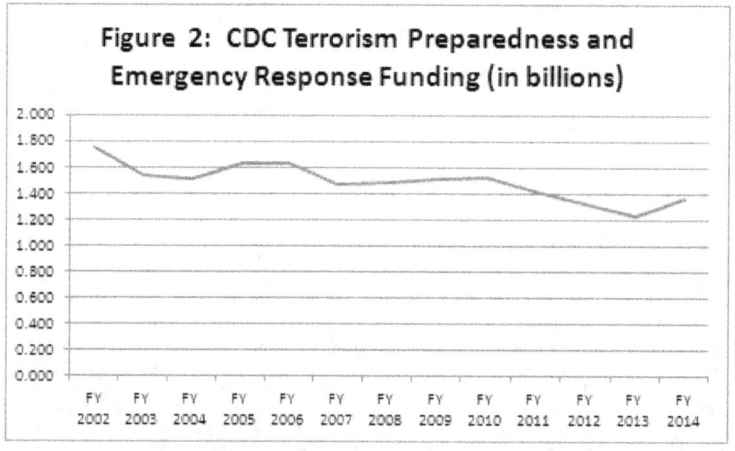

Figure 2: CDC Terrorism Preparedness and Emergency Response Funding (in billions)

This situation is also reflected at the State level. The Association of State and Territorial Health Officials (ASTHO) reported in September of this year that budget cuts continue to affect the health of Americans. Health departments in 48 States, three territories, and the District of Columbia have had budget cuts since 2008, with 95 percent of State or territorial health departments experiencing reduced services. Approximately 11,000 public health jobs have been lost in State health departments (*http://www.astho.org/budget-cuts-Sept-2014/*). The Trust for America's Health and Robert Wood Johnson Foundation released a report last December showing that the majority of States reached half or fewer of key indicators of policies and capabilities to protect against infectious disease threats. Texas scored 4 out of 10. One of the indicators (increased or maintained level of funding for public health services from fiscal years 2011–12 to fiscal years 2012–2013) was met by only 17 States (Texas was one of these 17 States), meaning that 33 States had decreased funding. Budgets in 20 States decreased 2 or more years in a row and 16 States had decreased budgets 3 or more years in a row (*http://healthyamericans.org/report/114/*).

Not unexpectedly, these trends in budget cuts can also be found at the local level. The National Association of County and City Health Officials (NACCHO) administers a biannual survey of local health departments (*http://www.naccho.org/topics/infrastructure/lhdbudget/upload/Survey-Findings-Brief-8-13-13-2.pdf*). Over 1 in 4 local health departments experienced a budget cut in the current fiscal year and, as shown in Figure 3, this has been an on-going declining trend.

Data from the 2013 survey show that the size of the public health workforce has decreased since 2008 when best estimates were 190,000 (range of 160,000 to 219,000) to 139,000 (range of 139,000 to 185,000), representing a total of 48,300 jobs lost. Almost half (41%) of local health departments Nation-wide experienced some type of reduction in workforce capacity, with, 48 percent of all local health departments reducing or eliminating services in at least one program area. Overall, State and local public health departments, the "boots on the ground" purveyors of public health, have lost over 51,000 jobs since 2008, representing one in five public health jobs.

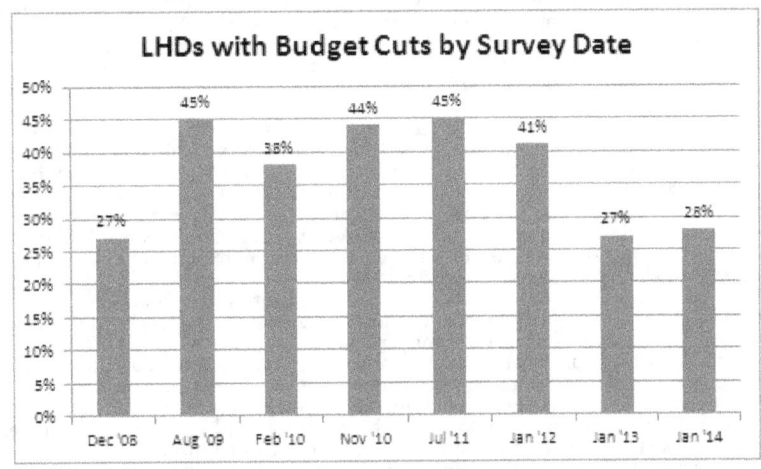

Now I'd like to put on my infectious disease expertise hat. The news coming out of West Africa is alarming. Almost 7,500 cases of Ebola with almost 3,500 deaths have been reported with many more suspected. Ebola is a frightening disease with horrific symptoms and concern is naturally high that further spread may occur. Is there a possibility that the next pandemic (defined as a world-wide epidemic) will be caused by Ebola? By looking at the characteristics of viruses that can spread world-wide, we can see that while there are some viruses capable of causing pandemics, Ebola is not one of them, and our undue anxiety over spread in the United States is diverting attention from true public health concerns.

Characteristics of a pandemic virus include:
• many people are susceptible to becoming infected;
• people can transmit the virus before they have symptoms;
• the virus causes severe symptoms and deaths;
• the virus is easily transmitted from person to person.

While Ebola has the first characteristic and certainly causes many deaths, it is lacking the two important ones—spread before symptoms occur and easy transmission. To become infected with Ebola, you must have physical contact with blood or bodily fluids from someone with symptoms. Unlike other viruses like influenza, people with Ebola are NOT infectious before symptoms appear. We know how to stop transmission by using barrier nursing practices such as gloves, disinfectants, and patient isolation. Unfortunately, many countries in Africa do not have the resources to provide for these precautions in their hospitals and so spread of Ebola is occurring in the health care setting. Adding to the problem are cultural practices where families prepare bodies of Ebola victims for burial, inadvertently becoming exposed to the virus. The conditions for spread of the Ebola virus in the United States and other resource-rich countries do not exist and the only danger is that we may be fixated on this virus and not on ones that could actually cause world-wide harm.

Given these characteristics, there are viruses that have outbreak or pandemic potential (or have caused these in the past) that public health agencies need to be on the look-out for—viruses such as influenza, SARS (severe acute respiratory syndrome), and MERS-CoV (Middle East Respiratory Syndrome), among others. Other "common" viruses such as measles and pertussis periodically cause outbreaks due to lack of immunity among those not vaccinated. Influenza is a virus that has caused pandemics in the past and has the potential to do so again. The virus can mutate so much that it's like a new virus no one has experienced before and so no one is immune. The great influenza pandemic of 1918 killed more people than World War I. There was concern in 2009 (when a new influenza virus appeared that looked like the 1918 virus) that we would again see a major influenza pandemic. While many people got infected, we were "lucky" that the virus did not kill more people than we typically see each flu season—although that number can be very high and the very young, seniors, and those with underlying illness are particularly susceptible. In Texas alone, over 2,300 people were hospitalized with 20 deaths in children last year. Many more were sick with the disease. Indeed, estimates are that up to 49,000 deaths occur Nation-wide each year due to seasonal influenza. Scientists are carefully monitoring some new influenza viruses that have been transmitted from birds to people, killing more than half of those infected, and although so far these avian flu viruses have not spread easily from person to person, the viruses could mutate to allow this to happen. Should this occur, a pandemic, with resultant high number of deaths, is almost inevitable.

MERS-CoV is caused by a virus currently occurring throughout countries in the Middle East. Although the disease spread through the air, as of right now, the virus does not appear to transmit easily from person to person (camels and/or bats are the most likely source of infection). While the chances of Ebola becoming airborne are exceedingly small (no pathogen has changed the way in which it is spread), it is more likely that small changes in the RNA of MERS-CoV could allow the virus to spread from person-to-person in a more efficient manner. Should this happen, the likelihood of a pandemic increases dramatically.

So what can we do to prepare for potential pandemics? Public health agencies such as CDC are constantly monitoring infections around the world to determine if new viruses are appearing. State and local health departments also are involved. Ebola virus is a major concern for the affected countries and the fear and loss of life are devastating on a humanitarian level. But we do not have to fear spread of the virus to the United States or other resource-rich countries. We would better spend our time preparing for diseases such as influenza which do have the potential to cause pandemics around the world, including the United States.

Congress must begin to prioritize public health funding and not just when a crisis occurs. Level or reduced funding for public health activities means that the same or less amount of money must cover prevention activities for an increased population. As recent outbreaks of food-borne illnesses, vaccine-preventable diseases, hospital-acquired infections, and emerging infectious diseases have shown, the threats remain and we need our public health community adequately funded to respond to these threats. While we are appreciative of the increased funding to combat Ebola contained in the recent continuing resolution signed by President Obama, an adequate response to the initial outbreak would have mitigated spread within Africa. According to a report by the Congressional Research Service, U.S. funding for World Health Organization (WHO) activities have decreased about one-third from 2010 to 2013. As seen in the U.S. public health system, this decreased funding resulted in WHO job losses and the ability to respond to emergencies such as Ebola.

Thank you for the opportunity to testify before you today about public health and our ability to deal with public health threats. I am happy to answer any questions you may have.

Chairman MCCAUL. Thank you, Doctor. The Chairman recognizes himself for questions.

Judge Jenkins, you mentioned that we have never encountered this before. I agree, this is new territory. In fact, in this county we experienced the first fatality due to Ebola in the United States. There is a lot of fear amongst not only residents here, but across the State and across America about this. We in Dallas County witnessed janitors wearing Tyvek suits in our schools. This really hits home.

So my question to Dr. Lakey and Dr. Giroir, what can you tell us here today, what can you tell the people of Dallas County, and the State of Texas, and the United States of America to alleviate these fears?

Dr. LAKEY. Thank you. I think the first thing, and I will repeat what I have already said, that we know the science. The CDC knows the science about this virus, that unless somebody is symptomatic, it is not contagious, that it is not spread in the air.

We are doing a lot of work right now to make sure that we do everything we can to prevent another Texan to be exposed to this virus. I believe this is a safe community. I feel safe enough. I have talked to the schools, I have talked to the emergency managers, I have talked to the hospitals, a wide variety of individuals and systems in Dallas and in Texas. One of the things that I told the schools, you know, I am a father. I would very comfortable with my kids going to these schools right now. They are not going to get Ebola from going to the schools right now.

We know the 48 individuals that had contact. We are monitoring them very closely. The kids that had contact, we are giving them home-based schooling to address this risk. But unless you have symptoms, you are not going to spread this disease. So, we take this very seriously. The monitoring is going very well, again, partners from the local level, the State level, the Federal level working together. Those 48 individuals that we are monitoring very closely, none of them are symptomatic.

Chairman McCAUL. Dr. Giroir, you have just been appointed the head of this task force. What are your plans to deal with this threat and deal with this fear amongst the population?

Dr. GIROIR. Well, first of all, I want to reiterate exactly what Dr. Lakey said, and I agree with every one of his points, that the transmission is, as he said, only by close contact with bodily fluids of an infected symptomatic person. Among the activities of this response, the ones that went very, very well were the identification of the contacts and institution of the appropriate monitoring. So we are very comfortable that that was done in a very effective and efficient way, and we will find ways to even improve on that even further. So all of these will be part.

One area that we will focus on in the task force is to make sure that all our potential notifiers really understand because a person with Ebola may not just walk into a major tertiary hospital. They may walk into their pharmacist, or they may walk into their local nurse, or their public health official.

So one thing we are going to have very, very early is a quick and rapid understanding to make sure we are educating all the potential people who could be the first contact with the patient, because the key to this whole success is identification of that patient and institution of monitoring, just like Dr. Lakey and the CDC team have done.

Chairman McCAUL. Dr. Giroir, in your testimony you mentioned there were issues involved in decontaminating the apartment in question, Mr. Duncan's apartment, including the needs for permits to transport the waste. Are you confident these issues have been resolved?

Dr. GIROIR. They were resolved. I am confident they have been resolved. A lot of it was by brute force and by working on issues as they came from the leadership that was there on the ground. What we want to do is make that much easier and much more facile the next time so that the leadership within the EOC can focus on the specific tasks at hand. Remember, next time it may not be 1 patient. It may be 5 patients, 10 patients with hundreds of contacts. So it was resolved effectively, but we have lessons learned. Maybe Dr. Lakey would want to comment on that.

Dr. LAKEY. I think that is right. This was a challenge, the first time you had to dispose of 140 55-gallon barrels, and they had to be put into another type of barrel, and have special permits from the Department of Transportation. I think we saw for this issue those barrels were burned today. They are gone, but I think this is an on-going issue we need to look at as a Nation. An event like this, how can we transport Class A medical waste and get rid of it quicker than what we could here in the State of Texas?

Chairman MCCAUL. Lastly, Dr. Giroir, you mentioned that this senior assistant for biodefense existed under both the Clinton and Bush administrations. I am not quite sure why that was eliminated under this administration. Is it, again, one of your recommendations that that position be reinstituted?

Dr. GIROIR. Again, I have no idea what are the reasons in the organization, but it is a strong recommendation that I have and a number of groups have for this position. You know, there is talk about Ebola czars or whatever, but this should not be a one-off. This should be a priority that transcends whatever disease is coming around the corner.

I know personally when I was at DARPA and the special assistant to the President called all the agencies in, all of a sudden it just was not a meeting where everybody had to have consensus and, you know, kind of figure out what everybody wanted to do and agree on the lowest common denominator. It was directives and leadership from someone who was in the White House.

I personally felt that made an enormous difference to organize our initial responses, whether that be in Africa or to write a pandemic flu plan. I personally feel, and I think you would get a lot of support, that that is the institutionalization at the highest level of a person responsible that you could turn to and we could depend on.

Chairman MCCAUL. So you knew who is in charge.

Dr. GIROIR. You knew who was in charge. The other comment is absolutely Health and Human Services has a huge part of this, but the Department of Defense also does. There are parallel programs. Homeland Security, as you know, identifies what is on the threat list that has to be transmitted. So this is bigger than one agency. There are 11 agencies funded in the biosecurity, biodefense areas, and there needs to be someone in charge. That is what this recommendation really is.

Chairman MCCAUL. Thank you. The Chairman recognizes the Ranking Member.

Ms. JACKSON LEE. Again, Mr. Chairman, let me thank you for this very important hearing, and let me thank my fellow Texans for setting a standard which the world can watch. Even as I pose these questions, it is at the backdrop of a great deal of thanks to all of you.

I wanted to just read just an excerpt from this morning's newspaper, which indicates that 6 U.S. military planes arrived in the Ebola hot zone. This article is making a statement in an article that Sierra Leone, as I indicated, they are pleading for our help. One of the African leaders said, "It is a tragedy unforeseen in modern times."

I do not want to, as I indicated, create hysteria. I want to be on alert. I think the important point to be made at this hearing for all of you is that all of those who may have been exposed will be watched and monitored for the full 21 days and maybe until the end of the month. Dr. Lakey, is that accurate?

Dr. LAKEY. We will be monitoring everyone exposed for the full 21 days.

Ms. JACKSON LEE. There are articles in the paper that indicate if they have not shown any signs in 10 days, then they are okay. I think that is a false premise that should be corrected by those who may perceive that. But you are saying that everyone will be monitored, is that correct?

Dr. LAKEY. All 48 contacts that we identified that have a risk of being infected with Ebola are being monitored daily. They have temperature checks twice a day. An epidemiologist sees them every day. I checked with them this morning. All of them are asymptomatic, yes.

Ms. JACKSON LEE. Let me thank Dr. Giroir. I did not indicate to you because one of my Baylor doctors and emergency doctors indicated that panels should be created across the Nation, so let me thank the State of Texas for creating that.

But let me make this point. As I indicated, six planeloads of our best and our brightest military personnel, they have to come home. I frankly do not believe that we are prepared, and I will tell you why. I ask the Chairman if I could submit into the record an article, "Even After Dallas, Hospitals Still Lagging Preparation for Ebola Patients, Say U.S. Nurses." I ask unanimous consent.

Chairman MCCAUL. Without objection, so ordered.*

Ms. JACKSON LEE. I particularly want to bring to your attention that one-third say their hospital has insufficient supplies of eye protection, feel shields, or side shields with goggles and fluid resistant impenetrable gowns. Dr. Lakey and Dr. Giroir, this is not condemnation. The CDC has done an amazing job. They are our theoreticians. They are the ones with theory and doing the research. But do we have a problem as we see the fluidness of people moving around the country, around the world, with making sure that every hospital that can afford the resources be prepared? Is that something that is necessary?

Dr. LAKEY. I will start, and then, Dr. Giroir, you can finish. I do not think preparedness is something you do and then you are done. You have to continue to work to be prepared. You have to continue to educate health care providers about exotic diseases and how do you respond to a major disaster.

---

*The information has been previously included in this document.

As I tell folks, unfortunately the unthinkable can happen. We are dealing with Ebola right now. While I have been in this chair I also responded to Hurricane Ike. We responded to H1N1, major events, and you have to have a strong public health system to do that. So, hospital preparedness funds and the other——

Ms. JACKSON LEE. So it would be important for us to make an assessment of whether equipment is in places where this may happen. I say that, Mr. Chairman, because an airplane was quarantined in Las Vegas just a few hours ago thinking there was an Ebola patient and it happened not to be. But ambulances and all, which is based upon people's fear, and that is what we need to do is to quell it, but we need to convince people that we are prepared.

Let me go quickly to Ms. Troisi on this funding situation. Do we need to ramp up our funding? Do we need to end the sequester? Would Medicaid be helpful here?

Ms. TROISI. I personally feel that, yes, we do need more funding for public health because as Dr. Lakey just said, public health is there all of the time. We should not be just be responding to crisis, and if you have a good system in place when a crisis does occur, you are better prepared.

Ms. JACKSON LEE. Medicaid expansion might help as well.

Ms. TROISI. Medicaid expansion would certainly help people who——

Ms. JACKSON LEE. I only have a few minutes. Thank you very——

Ms. TROISI [continuing]. Who do not have insurance.

Ms. JACKSON LEE. Thank you for your grace, Judge Jenkins, and your heart. We know how you lead in this county. Thank you for treating these individuals with dignity. But let me just say you expended dollars, 140 55-gallon barrels. What can we do to prepare for returning military personnel that may be all over America coming home as heroes, but having been in the hot spot of Ebola, and may, in fact, themselves be impacted coming to counties like Dallas County. What do you see that we would need to do in being prepared if that was to happen?

Judge JENKINS. Well, as far as the disease, the military I think has a good preparedness as people come home. It is very important to me that as our military men and women come home—Dallas County is the third choice in the country by popularity for them to return to—that we get them good jobs. You are on the right track that we need health care for people. We need Medicaid expansion. We need good jobs for our returning military.

The best thing that we can do to fight Ebola is to fight Ebola at its source overseas before it gets here.

Ms. JACKSON LEE. Thank you, Mr. Chairman. May I just add this to the record? It shows the kind of attire that should be used dealing with "Suiting up for Ebola." I ask unanimous consent to place this in the record.

Chairman MCCAUL. Without objection.

Ms. JACKSON LEE. I ask for these two documents, including "Ebola Outbreak Preparedness and Management," prepared by Doctors Without Borders*, to be put into the record.

Chairman MCCAUL. Without objection, so ordered.

[The information follows:]

Suiting up for Ebola

Some residents of West Africa are frightened by the protective suits worn by health workers aiding victims of the Ebola virus, but for those workers, personal protective equipment and strict disinfection procedures offer critical protection from the deadly disease, which is transmitted through contact with bodily fluids. Related article.

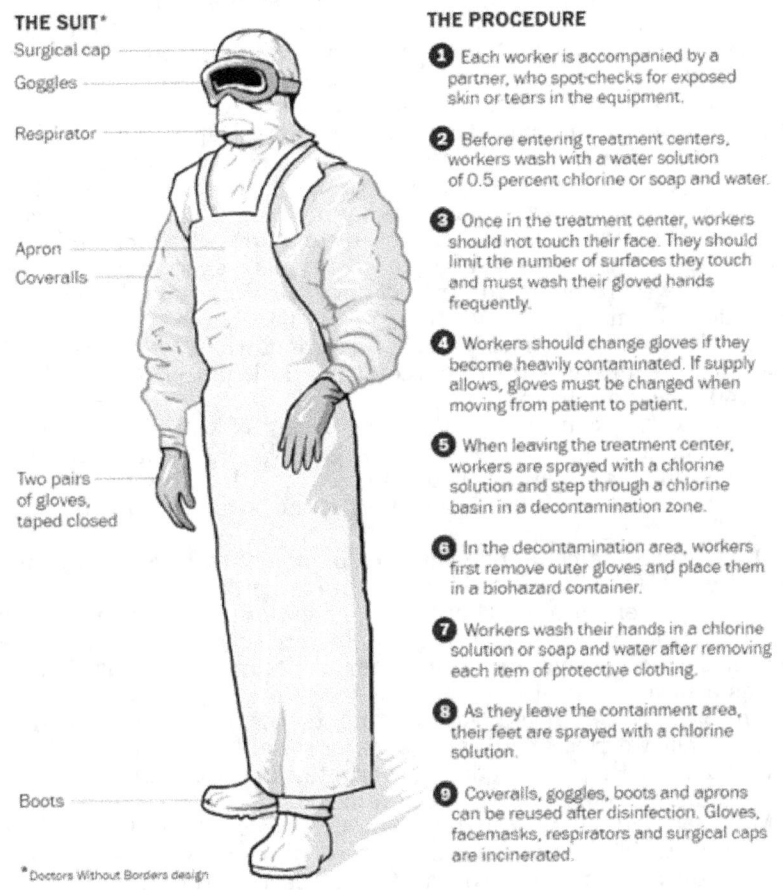

THE SUIT*

Surgical cap

Goggles

Respirator

Apron

Coveralls

Two pairs of gloves, taped closed

Boots

*Doctors Without Borders design

THE PROCEDURE

1 Each worker is accompanied by a partner, who spot-checks for exposed skin or tears in the equipment.

2 Before entering treatment centers, workers wash with a water solution of 0.5 percent chlorine or soap and water.

3 Once in the treatment center, workers should not touch their face. They should limit the number of surfaces they touch and must wash their gloved hands frequently.

4 Workers should change gloves if they become heavily contaminated. If supply allows, gloves must be changed when moving from patient to patient.

5 When leaving the treatment center, workers are sprayed with a chlorine solution and step through a chlorine basin in a decontamination zone.

6 In the decontamination area, workers first remove outer gloves and place them in a biohazard container.

7 Workers wash their hands in a chlorine solution or soap and water after removing each item of protective clothing.

8 As they leave the containment area, their feet are sprayed with a chlorine solution.

9 Coveralls, goggles, boots and aprons can be reused after disinfection. Gloves, facemasks, respirators and surgical caps are incinerated.

Ms. JACKSON LEE. I thank the gentleman.

Chairman MCCAUL. The Chairman recognizes the gentleman from South Carolina, Mr. Sanford.

---

*The information has been retained in committee files and is available at: *http://www.medbox.org/ebola/ebola-outbreak-preparedness-management/toolboxes/preview.*

Mr. SANFORD. Thank you, Mr. Chairman. Judge Jenkins, I do not know your story, but based on what I just heard, if you walked into an apartment with Ebola was there and somebody just died, I admire your courage, your humanity, your leadership in terms of just walking in without glove in hand, and shaking hands with folks, and giving them a hug as the case might have been. So I admire that.

But I want to go back to Dr. Lakey's comment. Well, in fact, everybody said the same thing. Everybody said you cannot get this disease unless it is from an infected party, a human contact. You are not going to get it out of the drapery over here. You are not going to get it out of the floor. You are not going to get it through the air, right? I mean, everybody has consistently said that.

Yet what we just heard was 140 55-gallon drums of hazardous waste were taken out of the apartment, which is to say unless the guy lived in a mansion, and I do not think he did, they flat-out stripped that apartment, in essence, down to the studs. I mean, they took out the carpet. They took out the drapes. They took out everything, threw it in. You had Class A hazardous material wherein you are having to fight permits in terms of getting it out.

Again, the folks back home are saying this does not connect for me. It is the same disconnect. We are told you are completely safe, but by the way, we are going to go to this guy's apartment that died, and we are going to strip it down to the studs. I mean, 140 55-gallon drums would fill this entire floor area right here. So which one is it? Is it really more hazardous than we think, or did they make a mistake in a degree of overkill, if you will, and drag out 140 55-gallon drums?

Dr. LAKEY. I can start, and then if any of the other panelists want to chime in. That would be great. We feel confident in the science that this is spread through contact with bodily fluids.

Mr. SANFORD. I understood that. Then why all the 55-gallon drums?

Dr. LAKEY. The challenge was in this apartment, you know, if he threw up, if there was other bodily fluids on curtains, et cetera, it had to be taken care of. There is a perception related to the apartment. You know, no one was going to rent that apartment unless you had done all you can do in order to decontaminate it. Because it was a Level A agent——

Mr. SANFORD. I mean, you are not in the real estate business. You are not worried about who is going to rent the apartment next.

Dr. LAKEY. But we needed to decontaminate the apartment, do everything we could to fully decontaminate——

Mr. SANFORD. Okay. But then you are going to the decontamination side, which is then it takes more than, as I have written it down, physical contact with an affected party. That is what is consistently said over and over and over again.

Dr. GIROIR. I think most of the leadership was concerned about blood, bodily fluids, other excretions that could have been in places in the apartment, such as in the bathroom, or rugs, or things like that. The data really show that the Ebola virus is very wimpy on surfaces, that it really goes away very quickly. It does not live very long at all. But if there is tissues, bodily fluids——

Mr. SANFORD. So, I mean——

Dr. GIROIR. So I believe there was a conscious decision to overly decontaminate and overly do waste removal because this was the first patient in the country. It was approached with an abundance of caution. For example, a toilet can be decontaminated, but do you want to sit there and decontaminate the toilet and have every question, or do just want to pick the toilet up, put it in a drum, and get rid of it, and be done? We had the luxury of only having one apartment to do, and I think with an abundance of caution——

Mr. SANFORD. Understood. Let me just follow up because I see I am down to a minute.

Dr. GIROIR. Yes, sorry.

Mr. SANFORD. The same question then in a different light in terms of the disconnect that I seem to be hearing from folks back home. A number of you all have talked about public health and the need to prioritize spending. We are well on our way to spending about a billion dollars in these three countries and sending in the military, which is a very expensive way of dealing with the problem. If, in fact, it is not as lethal and it could be handled by health care professionals rather than cranking up C–17s and sending them across the Atlantic, why not have health care professionals do it rather than $750 million, because we could then allocate some of the resources that Sheila Jackson Lee was just alluding or some of the other resources that are around the world given the crop up in Spain and other places?

Judge JENKINS. Sir, can I take a stab at that? It is extremely lethal. Fifty percent of the people in the world who get this disease die. The disconnect in what the visuals are on television is this. My contact and other officers' contact were with people who are being monitored to see if they become symptomatic. Their bodily fluids cannot transmit Ebola. The men in hazmat suits——

Mr. SANFORD. I understand that. I have run out of time, but I am still curious as to are we doing overkill then, spending a billion dollars with the military rather than having health care professionals. But I see I have run out of time, Mr. Chairman. Thank you, sir.

Chairman MCCAUL. Thank you, sir. The Chairman now recognizes Mr. Swalwell from California.

Mr. SWALWELL. Thank you, Chairman, and thank you to the officials for being here today, and thank you for what you are doing in this fight to keep Ebola from spreading here in the United States. I would just have to say just to follow up on my colleague from South Carolina, I certainly understand what he is saying, and I certainly understand, Dr. Giroir, the position that you are in and Dr. Lakey, which is on one hand if you have the case in America, people are watching it. We are in this Twitter, Facebook era where everything you do is going to be exponentially multiplied and told to the rest of the world.

But perhaps if the science is true that it can only be spread by direct bodily contact by somebody who is presenting the symptoms, if we are, as you said, Dr. Giroir, overly decontaminating, we could be our own worst enemy, and that by overly decontaminating, we are creating this perception that it is something that perhaps could be airborne.

So, I guess, my first question is, if you could just tell the public, you know, I will just go down the line, and each of you could pick one myth that you would like to dispel based on your expertise to the public, because my colleague from Texas, Congresswoman Jackson Lee, she is right. There is a plane right now in Vegas that people are just getting off because someone was coughing and sneezing, and people started freaking out and tweeting that they have Ebola. They were tweeting at Delta who was the carrier, and you can just imagine what that scene was like. So if I could just go down the line. One myth that you would like to dispel for the American public.

Dr. LAKEY. The first myth would be that the individuals that have been exposed but have no symptoms, that there is a risk. That is causing, I think, discrimination related to those individuals, and that is a myth that needs to be changed.

Mr. SWALWELL. Great, thank you. Dr. Giroir.

Dr. GIROIR. Again, just to reemphasize what everyone has said is that you have to be in close contact with the blood and body fluids of a person who is actively symptomatic. Again, if there were bodily fluids left on a carpet and you go there in a couple of hours, you know, there is a concern about that. But——

Mr. SWALWELL. Dr. Giroir——

Dr. GIROIR. Yes?

Mr. SWALWELL [continuing]. If Mr. Duncan had, as you said, perhaps thrown up in the apartment, how long would that bodily fluid be active, meaning if it was decontaminated, it was left there for days, weeks, months, how long would it be active?

Dr. GIROIR. Do you want to answer that?

Dr. LAKEY. I cannot tell you exactly how long it would be active in carpet. I cannot give you specific——

Ms. TROISI. There was a study just published. It was not specifically on carpet, but showing it lasts a couple of hours on surfaces at ambient temperature.

Mr. SWALWELL. Okay, thank you. Judge, how about a myth that you would like to dispel? You were right there on the front lines.

Judge JENKINS. Well, in the interest of repetition, and if people from the Dallas-Fort Worth area are watching, there is zero risk of you becoming infected from anyone who has come in contact with me or any first responder. We would never put your family and your children at risk. We follow CDC protocols. When we follow more than that, it causes panic.

Mr. SWALWELL. Ms. Troisi——

Dr. GIROIR. The task force does believe that there is significant opportunity to create less drums of waste moving forward. When you have an on-going relationship with a specific decontaminating contractor that you have set this up prospectively, that we do believe that there are really good opportunities to do less than was done. But on the first case in an acute situation, these situations were made by the incident command structure. I happened to be in the command post that day, but these were made by the incident commanders, and I fully support sort of the overabundance of caution in the first case.

Mr. SWALWELL. Thank you, Doctor. Ms. Troisi, if you had a myth you could dispel.

Ms. TROISI. Yes. Again, as everyone has said, Ebola is hard to get. You have to have direct contact. Whereas 1 person with measles typically infects 18 other people, with Ebola it is 2 other people.

Mr. SWALWELL. Thank you. So, Mr. Chairman, it sounds like to me, you know, fighting Ebola in West Africa has to be our primary goal, but also fighting myths at home just to prevent hysteria also has to be a priority. I yield back. Thank you.

Chairman MCCAUL. The Chairman now recognizes Mr. Clawson.

Mr. CLAWSON. Since I am from Florida, not from Texas, I would like to defer my time to Mr. Barton. I have got a question or two, but I will follow the Texans I think is the right way to go here.

Chairman MCCAUL. We admire that as Texans. Mr. Barton.

Mr. BARTON. Well, I appreciate my colleague from Florida. Today is my day to pick up my 9-year-old son from daycare, so I am very appreciative——

Mr. CLAWSON. That is a priority.

Mr. BARTON [continuing]. That I get to go next. Our first panel we focused on National and international issues, and my questions were directed primarily to why let people come into this region from the center of the disease, which is over in Africa. Well, this panel is a little bit different ball game. You have to deal with what is on the ground. It is not your issue how the people that might have the disease get into the United States. They are here. We have had a case here in Dallas, Texas, and the State of Texas has responded, Dallas County has responded. Some of the local hospitals have responded.

So my first question would be to you, Dr. Lakey. Dr. Merlin indicated that 114 people had been identified as having some significant contact with the individual who has since passed away from Ebola. Are you confident that your agency and CDC has everybody under observation who needs to be under observation?

Dr. LAKEY. Yes. I have talked to the CDC, the director here on the ground, and the other epidemiologist. They started out with 114, and then they took histories and talked to individuals, and they felt that those individuals, that there were 48. Now, I would say, yes, there are always rumors, and when there are rumors, we track them down to see if there is any truth to any of those rumors. That happens in every response.

But 48 individuals from all the analysis that the epidemiologists have had, the discussions linked with those individuals and with Mr. Duncan before he died indicated those 48 individuals, and those were the individuals that continue to be monitored. At the same time, I would say, yes, we are confident. We also understand that you always have to have a little humility when you are in a disaster. We prepare that if there was somebody else that was unreported, that we are ready for those individuals, too. So, that is my answer, sir.

Mr. BARTON. Do you have all the authority that you need to have to monitor, if necessary, quarantine and restrict individuals so that they do not transmit this disease to somebody else? Are there any restrictions on the State of Texas' Department of Health Authority to handle this situation?

Dr. LAKEY. This is one issue that I have been in the midst of, and I have the ability to put in a control order, and I put in three control orders. I do not take that lightly. I only did that because I had to ensure that we could monitor individuals effectively. If there was something that made me think that I could not do that, I put in a control order.

Now, my control order, though, is written documentation to that individual. It does not give the ability for the police to deter that individual. If the individual leaves, then you have to go get an Attorney General's opinion. The Attorney General Office goes to get a judge's opinion that then can give the ability for law enforcement to detain that individual.

Mr. BARTON. Is that the State of Texas Attorney General?

Dr. LAKEY. That is the State of Texas. So as I was discussing with some folks, I have more ability in my position to detain somebody for a short period related to mental health issues than I have with an infectious disease issue, like Ebola, initially because my order is written documentation, and only when they break that do I have the ability to get the police to detain that individual.

Mr. BARTON. So if Judge Jenkins, or the mayor of Dallas, or any other locally-elected official wanted to do something, they would come to you or your designee, and you would make the determination unless you felt it took a law enforcement action, which you would go to a district judge——

Dr. LAKEY. Yes, sir.

Mr. BARTON [continuing]. Who then would issue the proper authority for law enforcement to take whatever action you deem necessary.

Dr. LAKEY. The local health authority has that ability. This is a special situation, so I am here.

Mr. BARTON. So you are saying that the Dallas County Health Department has this authority. Either you have it, or they have it, or share it?

Dr. LAKEY. We both have it because we use it for tuberculosis, same type of control order. But that does not give us the power to detain until the individual breaks that control order. So you always have the possibility, and we have been doing this with putting the police out there so we do not lose an individual. But you have the ability that somebody could break that control order, and then you have to find them again.

Mr. BARTON. Now, how much longer do you have to monitor these 48 individuals before they are off the watch list and you can say with 99 percent confidence that there is no threat here in the DFW area, another 10 days?

Dr. LAKEY. We are monitoring them for 21 days. We are at day number 12 now.

Mr. BARTON. So 9 more days. If we do not develop a case, if they do not become symptomatic in the next 9 days, then we can safely say there is no danger immediately in the DFW area, is that correct?

Dr. LAKEY. That is correct. It gets a little bit complicated because the policies for overseas related to Ebola, they go two incubation periods, so 42 days. It is a little different situation since we know this one individual, but we will monitor the contacts for 21 days.

83

If there is anybody that was exposed, we monitor 21 days after that. So the individual patient, 21 days.

Mr. BARTON. I want to thank you, Mr. Chairman, for letting me participate. I also want to compliment the DFW Airport Authority for hosting this and putting it together so quickly. Finally, much has been made of the 140 barrels of hazardous waste material that has been collected and was incinerated today. The company that did that is in my Congressional district, and I want to commend that private-sector company for working with the local officials in such a conciliatory and cooperative fashion. They were willing to cut some of the red tape and so some things that needed to be done. With that, thank you for chairing this hearing and having it here in the DFW area.

Chairman McCAUL. It has been a real honor to have you, sir, and good luck with that 9-year-old boy.

[Laughter.]

Chairman McCAUL. The Chairman now recognizes the gentlelady from Texas, Ms. Eddie Bernice Johnson.

Ms. JOHNSON. Thank you very much, Mr. Chairman, and let me thank you for the hearing, and thanks to everyone who took the time to come today. I especially want to thank the panel. I cannot tell you how much appreciation I have for the type of leadership that you put into play when this happened. It could have been a lot worse. I am not certain it could have been much better, but I appreciate everything that you have done. I do not see anything that we left undone. I think that if there is a question, it might have been related to what happened between the first contact of the patient in the hospital, and that is not anything we are discussing today.

But what comes to mind is how well we can respond and how much we can over-respond sometimes if we do not use education and common sense and professionalism. Now, we have talked about stacking up a lot of equipment, goods, and supplies, which I think it is totally unnecessary. I do think we should be ready, but I also think we have to be concerned about expiration dates and how much we are stacking up for something that might not be necessary. So it does take some professional approach to determine what is going to be necessary to have a degree of readiness for any communicable disease.

We all are aware of the cuts. We all are aware that many of the cuts that we need to address. Sometimes we have overdone it. But I also want to remind everyone that when you ask for more airports to be added and more different other things to be added, that that is also another cost. So I just want you to know that when you ask for DFW to be included, I want to make sure that you include the budget for DFW to be included as well.

It is clear that we have dealt with and are dealing with a very serious disease that is affecting West Africa. We have done, I think, the best we could do with all of the anxiety that people experience with having one in this country. There are some other communicable diseases that are common in this country that we have not yet addressed quite as well, but we do have that ability.

But my caution is not to let our anxiety and the lack of clear education cause us to spend much more than what we need to. I went to the Department of Transportation to get permission for these goods to be disposed of, and I am delighted to be able to have done that. I do not know, and I cannot make a judgment at this point, how much was overdone or under done, but I think that I can be very clear in my appreciation to say that we did what we thought we needed to do for safety, for education, and to alleviate anxiety, and we will probably continue to do that. My caution is that we not overdo and over spend because we are still trying to address anxiety rather than the disease itself.

But at this point, I do not have any further questions, but just to express my appreciation to both the committee, the persons who came today, and to all of you who are on the front lines. And to say that I do not know anything else that I would have expected of our leadership from our Governor, to all of you who responded, to our local officials. I think that we did the best we could under the circumstances. It is a very new thing. I am not saying that we were perfect, but I am not sure that I can tell you what else you could have done. So thank you, Mr. Chairman, for having the hearing.

Chairman MCCAUL. Thank you as well. The Chairman recognizes Dr. Burgess.

Mr. BURGESS. Well, thank you, Mr. Chairman. This has been a very important afternoon, and I am certainly thankful that you let me participate. There will be another hearing on this subject next Thursday in Washington in the Energy and Commerce Committee. I spent the day yesterday in a field hearing in Raleigh-Durham on vaccine development. This is for people who think that we are not paying attention to this. I just want to underscore that.

I also just want to mention that I realize the CDC was on the previous panel, and it is easy to be critical of the Federal agencies. But I would also say that it is the CDC that goes afield and does the work. Yes, the World Health Organization is there, but I will tell you the global outreach and resource network of the World Health Organization would be nothing without the participation of the CDC. They have borne the lion's share of this burden overseas and in the United States. The United States taxpayer has borne the lion's share of this burden, and I do hope that other global partners will step up because fighting the disease, you know, on the fronts in Africa is extremely important.

We were told by all the experts that this would burn itself out, March/April time frame, and then when it did not, of course it was so much more established that it is now. As I pointed out on Mr. Thompson's graph, were are in the exponential phrase. It is very, very difficult to control a disease in the exponential phase.

But we have also, I think, lost an opportunity here at home to provide that public trust or that public confidence, and that is going to be hard to get back, and that is why so much of the discussion that you heard with the earlier panel dealt with how do we deal with people coming in. Okay, no direct flights. It turns out there are 125, 150 people a day who come from those countries in Africa to this country. Perhaps we should increase the surveillance period. Yes, that would cost some additional money, but, you know, it is the old deal, a stitch in time saves nine.

We are paying an enormous amount of money for the fact that someone got through, the problem has happened, and then the whole cascade. Then as a consequence to that, and, Dr. Lakey, you and I discussed this, I mean, this problem does not stop at the county line. One of your employees, Judge Jenkins, one of my constituents, who had a problem the other day, and once that threshold is reached again, the entire cascade has to happen yet again with all of the concern and all of the expense.

Dr. Giroir, I would be interested in your thoughts because you have participated at the Federal level before. Is there not something more we can do at the beginning phase of this when people are coming into this country to hold people a little longer, to keep a little tighter surveillance, and not have to bear the expense at Judge Jenkins' level and Dr. Lakey's level?

Dr. GIROIR. Again, international travel is really not my area of expertise, but I do want to underscore as in any situation like this, the further you push this event to the left, the better you are going to be. So the earlier you identify the individual, if that is going to be in the hospital in the emergency room that first time or when they go to the pharmacist, that first identification is very important.

The earlier you do that and the further you push that back, that is where it needs to be done because by the time you close down a 24-bed ICU, you activate all of the EOCs, that is really not the way you want to attack this. It would be great——

Mr. BURGESS. It is the most expensive way.

Dr. GIROIR. It is the most expensive and the least effective way. So you get it at its origin in Africa, this disease in Africa. There will be other diseases in other parts of the world, and maybe we will originate some that the other parts of the world will deal with as well. It is not an African issue. It is a world issue. But again, I agree with what you said. You get it as close to the source as possible. You do not try to play catch-up once it is here and it is out.

Mr. BURGESS. Dr. Lakey, you referenced an after-action report. I referenced that in my earlier discussion with the earlier panel. Is there actually a report that is going to be produced by the State?

Dr. LAKEY. We do that after every major event. We did it after H1N1. We did it after Hurricane Ike. It is part of our policy. We are a learning agency, and we have to learn from our experience. So, yes, we do an after-action after every major event.

Mr. BURGESS. Well, I am sure Mr. McCaul would like you to share that with the Homeland Security Committee. I would just ask that we just share that with the Energy and Commerce Committee as well.

Dr. LAKEY. Absolutely.

Mr. BURGESS. Then, Judge Jenkins, finally, again, your employee, my constituent, who had a problem the other day, and not to get into the details or specifics of that. But is there a contact number that someone has who might have a concern about this who was in that, not the primary group, the 48 people that you are talking about, but in, say, a secondary or even a tertiary group where they can talk with someone before having to pull the lever of going to an urgent care center or an emergency room. Is there an intake place that they have available to them?

Judge JENKINS. There is, and your constituent and my employee, I spoke to him this morning, and I spoke to his wife, and I spoke to the head of his association. What I told him is that he has my full support. He and his family acted appropriately on the information they were given by someone outside. They were given information that we were unaware of at the incident command structure, and they acted on that.

The information within the incident command structure would be different, and we have had a meeting now with all law enforcement at the agency level, at the association level, to let them speak to infectious disease doctors from the other Dallas area hospitals that are unaffiliated with the Government or Presbyterian Hospital and get their questions answered. We have set up a location for them to receive care should they have any sorts of concern.

But let me make something very clear to the public. There is a 0 percent chance that I or my deputies or my first responders contracted Ebola because I and my deputies and my first responders did not come into contact with any bodily fluids of Mr. Duncan.

Mr. BURGESS. I appreciate that. I do hope that this information will part of that after-action report as it is all incorporated when you look back at the entire series of events.

Judge JENKINS. Congressman, I also want to stress that we want a complete after-action. To the extent permitted by law, I want that to be public.

Mr. BURGESS. Yes, I agree. Thank you, Mr. Chairman. Thank you for holding the hearing.

Chairman MCCAUL. Thank you, Doctor, for your expertise. The Chairman recognizes Ms. Jackson Lee for the purpose of introduction of a document into the record.

Ms. JACKSON LEE. Let me thank you, Mr. Chairman. I would like to add into the record a letter dated October 8, 2014 officially requesting for the enhanced screening and CDC at Bush Intercontinental, and I would add that I join on DFW as well. Let me conclude, Mr. Chairman. I know there is one more, I think, testimony coming. Two more. Just to say that I want to thank all these gentleman. I am stepping away for an airplane. I want to give my appreciation and thanks, and I want to thank Commissioner Jenkins for, again, your grace and humanity.

To the others, I will put into the record, Mr. Chairman, my question about contagion units as well as my question regarding the idea of the panels that the Governor was astute in putting in this State, whether they would be appropriate. Again, this hearing is not just for Ebola, but to be prepared for any episode that we might come in contact with, and I thank the witnesses very, very much. I thank this community very, very much. I yield back.

Chairman MCCAUL. Without objection, so ordered with respect to the document.

[The information follows:]

October 8, 2014.

Dr. Tom Frieden,
Director, Centers for Disease Control and Prevention, 1600 Clifton Road—Mailstop E–92, Atlanta, GA 30329–4027.

Dear Dr. Frieden: As a Senior Member of the House Committee on Homeland Security and the Ranking Member of the Subcommittee on Border Security, I am pleased that the Centers for Disease Control, the Department of Homeland Security's U.S. Customs and Border Protection Agency, and the United States Coast Guard are coordinating to establish a new level of screening for international air travelers during the global Ebola health crisis that is impacting the United States. I understand this coordinated effort will add new screening protocols beginning Saturday, October 11, 2014 for passengers with flight itineraries where travel originated in the countries of Guinea, Liberia, or Sierra Leone. Additionally, I am aware that the Centers for Disease Control and the Department of Homeland Security announced new layers of entry screening at Hartsfield-Jackson Atlanta International Airport, Newark Liberty International Airport, John F. Kennedy International Airport, Dulles International Airport, and Chicago O'Hare International Airport.

As a Member of Congress representing, Houston Texas, the 4th largest city in the nation, I am requesting that George Bush Intercontinental Airport be included on the list of airports to receive the enhanced Ebola screening protocols for those passengers whose flight itineraries indicate that the air travel originated in the countries of Guinea, Liberia, or Sierra Leone. The George Bush Intercontinental Airport serves the Houston area and is a major originating and connecting hub for international air travelers. From January to August 2014, there have been 99,452 West African passengers traveling into and out of the George Bush Intercontinental Airport with a total of 1,856,421 international travelers. I am requesting that George Bush Intercontinental Airport be added to the list of airports receiving new layers of entry screening.

The new layers of entry screening that should be followed at the George Bush Intercontinental airport include: (1) Customs and Border Protection agents greeting passengers and escorting them to a quarantine area where they will answer questions from a detailed questionnaire; (2) United States Coast Guard trained medical staff conducting a preliminary health screening by checking temperatures with a contact free thermometer; and (3) Centers for Disease Control staff making further health assessments to determine whether a passenger should go to a hospital. Further, these passengers will be provided with information on signs of the illness and information on self-quarantine and who to contact for medical assistance. If a passenger's answers to the questionnaire indicate that future follow up and tracking should be done, they will referred to a county health department for follow up medical assessment.

I am available to speak with you regarding the George Bush Intercontinental Airport and the status of their level of preparedness as well as the hospitals and first line health care providers serving the city of Houston.

Very truly yours,

Sheila Jackson Lee,
Member of Congress.

Chairman McCaul. Mr. Clawson is recognized.

Mr. Clawson. Thank you for your service. Thanks for coming here today. I am not from Texas, but I can see you all are very competent in what you do and very knowledgeable, and I am very appreciative for you coming here today.

A few years ago I got off a plane from India for my business. It was the monsoon season, and there were big dang mosquitoes everywhere. About a week later in the United States I became very ill with a hemorrhagic illness and went to the hospital, and was ordered tested for malaria and a few other things, but was not tested for chikungunya for that matter or any of the other illnesses that, by the way, are getting closer and closer to our country and to Texas.

So when the incident happened in Texas, I really was not surprised because just from my own experience, it seemed to me that this idea that the folks in our emergency rooms could have enough first-hand knowledge of the different hemorrhagic infectious diseases around the world and match them with the travelers. I had told my doctor that I was coming from India, and it was the monsoon season. It feels like a really hard task that you are up against because the first line has got to be 100 percent, and it is a complicated world.

So I draw two conclusions or questions from that. How do we get that knowledge at the hospital level really ingrained, and second, whatever you all are learning here because you are on a steep learning curve, right? How do we get it to other States and areas like mine so that we do not have to re-learn tough lessons? Will you all respond to that a little bit?

Dr. LAKEY. I will start, and then I will hand off. I think you are right. I think we have to be prepared for the next event. I would not be surprised if we have something like this somewhere else in the United States. We were just unfortunate here in Texas.

I think a lot of the things that you saw happen here could happen in other places with somebody not fully understanding the travel history, not making the link of what is going on halfway around the world, and making the first diagnosis of a tropical disease here in the United States. So we have to learn from one another.

So some of those things that we do, there is an organization of the folks that do my job across the United States. We have had multiple phone calls related to this strategic plan issue, chikungunya, et cetera, and we share information rapidly between each other. There is a Council of Epidemiologists across the United States. They have had those types of meetings. We have to educate here in the State of Texas. We have had multiple phone calls with all the hospitals, all the EMS providers, all the emergency managers across the State of Texas. We will share our after-action report and share that information with our colleagues across the United States. But we take that very seriously.

I think also to reiterate some of the comments that were made earlier, I do not think you ever get done with preparedness. So, those funding streams for hospitals to be prepared or for public health emergency preparedness really are essential for hospitals, for clinicians, for public health individuals across the United States so they know how to recognize when something like this occurs and have the expertise to respond quickly. Those funds have been reduced over the last several years, and they are essential to a health department like mine to be able to respond effectively to an event like this.

I guess the other thing I would add is that many years ago there were dollars that went to academic institutions to provide disaster education, and those funds have also been decreased over the last several years.

Dr. GIROIR. It is always very difficult for a low-risk, high-consequence event to have everyone thinking about those events. After you have the first event, everybody is thinking about those events. We have done this in the past with the college meningitis. There was a big outbreak in North Texas, and the mortality rate went down many-fold just by education, but it is not just education. It is really getting on the ground and making sure people understand how to act on that education.

I can say our task force, we can say all the good things, but you do not know until you ask the people who are on the front line. So we have a formal process we will be announcing to seek information from the Texas Medical Association, Nurses Association, Pharmacy Association, Public Health Association, the first responders, the Rural and Community Health Association, because not everybody lives in an urban area. We are a rural State.

So we want to seek a lot of input in how we could best educate the diverse groups and make that on-going. It may be as simple as, I do not know if this is simple or effective, but we all have continuing medical education, you know, 24 hours every 2 years. Have 15 minutes, just a 15-minute on-line that it does not matter whether you are a nurse, a doctor, or a pharmacist, that says what is circulating—what do you need to worry about? It takes 15 minutes, and at least you reach everybody during that basis. But we will be exploring all those efforts.

Mr. CLAWSON. Well, let us hope that we can get everybody in the country in those jobs having that 15 minutes, right, because it seems like a pretty important 15 minutes.

Dr. GIROIR. Yes, sir.

Judge JENKINS. Can I answer that from the perspective of what you could take home to your local governments for them to do immediately?

Mr. CLAWSON. It would be very helpful.

Judge JENKINS. Yes, sir. Every county that you represent needs to have a protocol for identifying people who have recently traveled to West Africa and have certain symptoms, and then quarantine them into a private room, and take appropriate precautions. We had that in Dallas County. It was not followed in this case.

At some hospitals, the electronic medical records have artificial intelligence that would trigger that. That would be a good best practice for large hospitals. The incident command in a box for Ebola, that is not just a game plan. You have actually contacted those cleaning guys and those apartment or home residences you are going to move people to, and they are actually going to clean up after Ebola, and actually going to take contact families into their premises. There is going to be a security perimeter around that to keep out onlookers.

Where we fell down is not that David and I could not white board what needed to happen. It was the length of time it took to make it happen, and it took a phone call from me to a member of the faith community after we exhausted every housing source in Dallas County, 2.5 million people. It took a call to the faith community and asking them to clear out an area and do this for us, and that is not any way to have to do this.

Chairman MCCAUL. Thank you. The Chairman recognizes Mr. Farenthold.

Mr. FARENTHOLD. Thank you very much, Mr. Chairman. You did a great job of getting a bipartisan panel. We have an Aggie and somebody from The University of Texas here.

[Laughter.]

Mr. FARENTHOLD. So we have a great bipartisan panel.

Chairman MCCAUL. I am going to stay out of that one.

Mr. FARENTHOLD. Mr. Jenkins, I want to follow up on what Mr. Clawson was asking. You know, listen, yes, I think you did a phenomenal job, the humanity that you showed, and I join you in my sympathy for Mr. Duncan's family. But my question is, you talked a little bit about what all the counties need to be doing, actually having the places. Can you take maybe a minute-and-a-half and just give me your top 5 things that the county judges and all the other Texas counties ought to be thinking about and doing?

Judge JENKINS. You need to make sure you have protocols and that our hospitals have been training with repetition. You need to activate your medical societies so that they are training with that repetition and interactions with your hospitals. Then on your instant command in a box, you need to have that laid out and ready to go on a moment's notice.

You need to have places for people to move to, people to clean things up. Your first responders need to know what the protocols are to handle these situations. You need to have a messaging plan to keep people calm and have them follow the science. You need to bring in your schools early and your faith community early and help them be messengers. You need to empower all of your school boards, your city councils in your suburban areas. You need to do that in the first 24 hours.

Mr. FARENTHOLD. All right. Mr. Giroir, we have heard a lot about the failure of this information to get down to the front-line folks in the hospital. I mean, that was kind of the big screw-up here I think. I get hundreds of emails every day. I used to be a computer guy. I would get somebody from the Computer Emergency Response Team. I get all sorts of information like that in my inbox. When I have got a busy day, that just is the first thing that does not get read are the, you know, the emails with important updates.

You talk about a 15-minute continuing medical education, 15 minutes every 2 years. Does not this change more than every 2 years? I mean, that probably would not be enough. I mean——

Dr. GIROIR. No, it certainly would not.

Mr. FARENTHOLD. How do you get around that? I mean, everybody knows about Ebola if they have turned on their television newscasts now. But what happens early on when the next one comes?

Dr. GIROIR. Right, and I think you are exactly right. We do not know if the information did not get to the people in the emergency room or they did not act on the information in the correct way. That will be something in the future.

But you are correct that the best way to approach any problem, and you do it in hospitals all the time, is to create processes that you cannot get around. As the judge said, the Texas Senate heard testimony of one of the large hospitals, Parkland, where it is an automated record that if you are from West Africa, it literally lights up on every screen, and it has to go to a higher-level supervisor in order to make sure that it is appropriately handled. Those kinds of fail-safe mechanisms do not rely on individual emails or education, but it is a multifaceted approach.

Mr. FARENTHOLD. How do you get away from the reluctance? Again, I am an old computer guy. There is nobody who hates computers more than doctors. I mean, every doctor I know has complained about electronic medical records and the expert systems.

Dr. GIROIR. But we do educate providers. We do keep them up. There are continuing medical educations. There are conferences. There are meetings. There are other ways to reach people. But there is no single solution. This is going to be a comprehensive education solution that spans many, many disciplines because, again, not everybody goes to a hospital ER. They may show up at a pharmacist, or a public health professional, or a nurse, or from promotoras in the colonias. We have to have this widespread. It is a challenge, there is no doubt.

Mr. FARENTHOLD. All right. Finally, I think everybody on the panel has said that funding needs to be restored for a variety of projects. What else can we do as Congress to help with this beyond kicking up the budgets? Is there legislation we need to do? Are there holes? What else is there to do besides spend some more money? Go ahead, Judge.

Judge JENKINS. Streamline the process for permitting for waste. Empower public health officials and executives. I serve as the director of homeland security and emergency management for Dallas County. Give us the power to do this quicker. We are working under laws that clearly were not set up for Ebola.

Mr. FARENTHOLD. Anybody else?

Dr. LAKEY. I would agree. I talked a little bit about the ability of a health authority to be able to detain an individual, understanding that you do not want that to be very broad, an emergent issue, to be able to do this. We talked about funding. The health alert networks, the basic abilities to do surveillance activities, monitor individuals, having exercises that take place in hospitals, the requirements for continuing medical education, those types of things.

I guess the other idea that I would have is I was able to participate this summer with the Institute of Medicine looking at how we can we improve the ability to do research in the middle of a disaster. I think you need to think about how can we facilitate that in an emergent event to rapidly be able to take investigational drugs, to monitor them appropriately, and to decrease that time that it took to get research done and investigational medicines out.

Mr. FARENTHOLD. I see, Ms. Troisi, you look like you want to answer.

Ms. TROISI. Yes, really.

Mr. FARENTHOLD. I do not have a lot of time, but if the Chairman will——

Ms. TROISI. No, I will add one thing, is that disease-specific funding hampers public health's ability to prioritize what needs to be done. Many times communities that have one problem have another problem, but the funding streams are such that you can only deal with problem A, not with problem B with that specific funding. So non-restricted funds would be good.

Mr. FARENTHOLD. Thank you very much.

Dr. GIROIR. Money is important, but accountability for the funds, money spent right, is equally as important as the amount of money, and that takes leadership across agencies. I think there is tremendous duplication even in my area between DoD and DHHS that could be easily streamlined for less money.

The third thing I would say, and I am on the other side of this now, is that probably the onerous Government contracting procedures probably double the time and increase the costs by 30 or 40 percent than what they need to be. Congress has given special contracting authorities to certain agencies to allow that to be expedited, and they are not being expedited in their fullest. We can get more for the money we spend right now.

Mr. FARENTHOLD. Thank you.

Chairman MCCAUL. We thank the witnesses for this hearing, for being here. It has been very informative, and not only in terms of identifying the threat and how to best contain and control it, but also to debunk some of these myths out there in terms of Ebola and how it is transmitted. I think that will go a long way in alleviating some of the panic and the fears out there in the general population.

So the record will stay open for 10 days. Members may have additional questions to submit in writing.

With that, Ms. Jackson Lee is recognized.

Ms. JACKSON LEE. Thank you so very much. On behalf of Mr. Thompson, I want to also express my appreciation to the Chairman and to all of you. I think in addition to debunking, I think there has been given comfort that health professionals across America, we cannot have hearings with every county and State, but that there is a preparedness and a readiness to be prepared, and the recognition that we may not have rural hospitals before us.

Texas Presbyterian may be the one in the eye of the storm and people are looking into how that treatment was. But at least you have given a pathway for our hospitals and medical facilities to reach out for information, to determine if they have the right amount of equipment, and as well, to raise questions such as the kind of containment units.

Again, I am going to push this idea of regional panels. Dr. Giroir, I think it is an excellent idea, and we have learned a lot from hearing what Texas has done. Thank you all so very much. Thank you, Dr. Lakey——

Chairman MCCAUL. With that, the committee is adjourned.

[Whereupon, at 4:01 p.m., the committee was adjourned.]

APPENDIX

Question 1. In understanding that there may be some accuracy questions or concerns around reliance on a non-contact thermal thermometer, what steps will the CDC or other agencies take to achieve secondary/confirmatory screening to ensure optimal accuracy and quality and potentially more precision in readings?

Answer. Response was not received at the time of publication.

Question 2. Could you provide the committee with background on the decision process that went into the choice of the thermometer(s) that will be utilized?

Answer. Response was not received at the time of publication.

Question 3. Will the temperature screeners be maintaining the recommended distance barrier (3 ft.) for evaluation and if so, how will they use the infrared devices effectively?

Answer. Response was not received at the time of publication.

Question 1a. The Center for Disease Control and Prevention (CDC) provides grant funding to ensure that public health departments are prepared for emergencies. What are the audit and accountability mechanisms for CDC Public Health Emergency Preparedness (PHEP) grants?

Was any of the PHEP funding spent in Texas and specifically in Dallas?

Question 1b. If so, how was this funding spent and why did this not prevent the mistakes that occurred in Mr. Eric Duncan's case?

Question 1c. Given the public health errors made in Dallas with regards to Mr. Duncan's case, what procedural changes does CDC recommend?

Answer. Response was not received at the time of publication.

Question 2a. There was a 4-day delay from when Mr. Duncan was diagnosed and when he received the experimental treatment. What effect did this have on Mr. Duncan's death?

I understand that CDC cannot mandate the specific type of care, but what are your thoughts on the efficacy of the treatment Mr. Duncan received?

Question 2b. Was the hospital adequately prepared?

Answer. Response was not received at the time of publication.

Question 1. Dr. Merlin, at the October 10 hearing I asked you about the budget of the Centers for Disease Control and Prevention (CDC). I inquired if the CDC's budget was adequate or if it needed to be increased. And, I asked what would be done with this additional funding if it were needed. You answered that you would defer to the CDC director and Department of Health and Human Services (HHS). Having had time now to consult with the director of the CDC and anyone at HHS, how would you answer my questions about the adequacy of the CDC's budget and what would be done with extra funds if they were considered needed?

Answer. Response was not received at the time of publication.

Question 2a. I followed up my question about the general CDC budget with a question about the budget of just your part of CDC, the Division of Preparedness and Emerging Infection. You said you would have to get back to me. Please now provide information about the budget of the Division of Preparedness and Emerging Infections. Specifically, include the level of funding your division has received between fiscal year 2005 and fiscal year 2015. Please also note the effect of sequestration.

Do you consider these levels of funding adequate to accomplish your mission?

Question 2b. If not, what have been the negative effects of these insufficient amounts?

Answer. Response was not received at the time of publication.

Question 3a. Dr. Francis Collins, head of the National Institutes of Health (NIH), recently said the following in talking about the impact of budget cuts on finding a vaccine for Ebola: "Frankly, if we had not gone through our 10-year slide in research support, we probably would have had a vaccine in time for this that would've gone through clinical trials and would have been ready."

Do you share Dr. Collins's view?

Question 3b. Why or why not?

Answer. Response was not received at the time of publication.

QUESTION FROM HONORABLE LAMAR SMITH FOR JOHN P. WAGNER

Question. What type of precautions will the involved agencies be taking to protect the screeners at the airport (i.e. will they all use personal protective equipment (PPE) to include gloves, surgical masks). And if so, will that differ from the precautions they plan to take for the screeners of those passengers who have an elevated temperature?

Answer. U.S. Customs and Border Protection (CBP) Office of Field Operations (OFO) has received guidance from the Department of Homeland Security (DHS) Office of Health Affairs (OHA) and Centers for Disease Control and Prevention (CDC) on Ebola entry screening and the requirements for the use of Personal Protective Equipment (PPE) for enhanced Ebola screening. OFO has distributed this guidance to the CBP employees at the ports of entry (POE) processing international travelers arriving from or transiting through the countries affected by the Ebola virus outbreak.

DHS guidance on Ebola entry screening outlines the requirements of PPE use, including proper procedures for putting on (donning), taking off (doffing), and wearing PPE. DHS guidance outlines the required PPE that must be worn when an employee is in close proximity to a traveler from a country of concern. In addition, the guidance outlines the additional required PPE to be worn by an employee when working in close proximity to a traveler from a country of concern who is exhibiting symptoms consistent with the Ebola virus.

PPE has been made available to all CBP employees at the five designated POEs where enhanced Ebola screening is being conducted along with OHA guidance which includes the Job Hazard Analysis and PPE Assessment. CBP has deployed formal training to CBP employees conducting enhanced screening on the donning and doffing of PPE and will be implementing additional training on PPE and enhanced screening protocols.

CBP is in the process of deploying additional PPE to all POEs, and all POEs have been instructed to maintain a 60-day supply of PPE at each location.

○